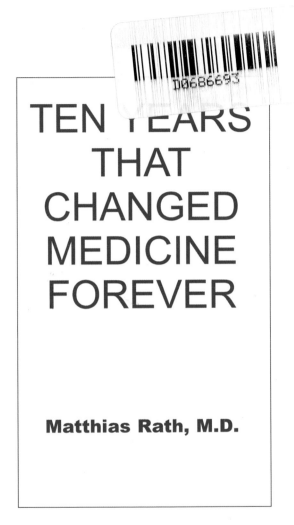

TEN YEARS THAT CHANGED MEDICINE FOREVER

Matthias Rath, M.D.

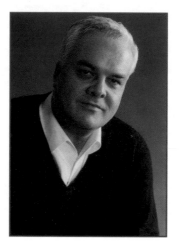

Matthias Rath, M.D.

© 2001 Matthias Rath, M.D.
ISBN 0-9679546-3-0

MR Publishing Inc.
4699 Old Ironsides Drive
Suite 300
Santa Clara, CA 95054

www.dr-rath-research.org

RSA00004

Contents

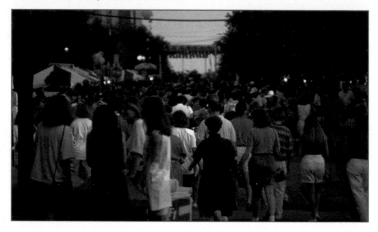

This book is dedicated to the six billion people living today and to the generations of our children and grandchildren.

INTRODUCTION

*"We had suffered, starved and triumphed,
grown bigger in the bigness of the whole.
We had reached the naked soul of man."*
Sir Ernest Shackelton, Polar explorer, 1908

Two-time Nobel Laureate Linus Pauling stated that Dr. Rath's discoveries will be seen as the most important revelations of the second half of the 20th century. This book tells the story.

Never before has a medical breakthrough so directly and immediately affected the lives of millions of people. This book explains the consequences of these discoveries for millions of patients.

David Against Goliath

Never before has the medical truth been fought so fiercely by a multi-billion-dollar industry, the pharmaceutical industry, whose very basis is the "business with disease." This is the war diary of this battle.

Never before has a David-Goliath confrontation so heavily depended on one man to resolve a problem for the benefit of millions of people. This is the account of the scientist who forced the pharmaceutical Goliaths to accept the scientific truth and embark on large-scale vitamin research.

The last decade of the twentieth century will go into the records of history as the period when the pharmaceutical companies multi-billion-dollar "business with disease" was turned into a "business towards health," a monumental step in human history and the precondition to the ultimate stage, when good health will become a human right.

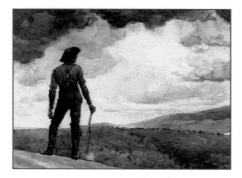

Triggering the Vitamin-Cartel

Ten years ago, large pharmaceutical companies, including Roche, BASF and Archer Daniels Midland, formed a vitamin cartel and conspired to fix the price of vitamin raw materials. These criminal actions artificially raised the price of vitamins for every household in America, Europe and beyond.

While these companies paid billions of dollars in fines, no one has asked the most important question of all: What triggered the pharmaceutical giant's actions? A multi-billion dollar price-fixing conspiracy reflects expectations of a growing consumer demand for these vitamins. This book describes how Dr. Rath informed Hoffman-LaRoche about the medical breakthrough that triggered some of the largest pharmaceutical companies in the world to become involved in criminal activities.

Fighting the Pharmaceutical Cartel

This book also explains the background of one of the great victories for human health in America: The Dietary Supplement Health and Education Act (DSHEA) of 1994. This "Vitamin Freedom Act" was the answer of the American people to a two year campaign by the American pharmaceutical companies and the FDA to make vitamins prescription items.

Again, no one asked the most important question: What triggered this unethical effort? Why did the pharmaceutical companies want to make vitamins prescription items - against the will of over 100 million vitamin consumers? This campaign by the pharmaceutical companies and the FDA is not an action but a reaction to a scientific discovery that threatened a multi-billion-dollar market in cardiovascular prescription drugs. This book documents the background of this campaign in the inter-est of the multi-billion dollar "business with disease."

Did you know that there is a United Nations commission called *Codex Alimentarius* (regulation for nutrition) that has been trying since 1996 to outlaw vitamin therapies on a worldwide scale? This book tells how thousands of patients whom Dr. Rath had already helped came to Berlin in June 2000 and succeeded in stopping these unethical global plans.

Turning Nutritional Medicine Into Established Medicine

Read how pharmaceutical giants were forced to enter the vitamin research field. Within eight weeks after this historic defeat, Hoffman LaRoche announced that they would establish an independent vitamin research subsidiary. BASF - one of the companies spearheading the unethical *Codex* plans - was buying Takeda, the second largest manufacturer of vitamin C.

With the global players forced together and substantiating health benefits of vitamins on a large scale, nutritional medicine will become established medicine within the next decade. With this encouraging development foreseeable, new challenges arise.

Nutritional health and medicine must not fall into the hands of a monopoly. All mankind must share nutritional health.

Receiving the Torch from Linus Pauling

This book breathes history. Join Dr. Rath as he talks about his close relationship with the late Nobel Laureate Linus Pauling, who saw in him his successor. Witness the interests they shared in science and vitamin research, the joint zeal of these two scientists for making good health a human right and contributing to a better world.

Join them at their historic press conference at the Mark Hopkins Hotel in 1992. In Linus Pauling's last public appeal, the Nobel Laureate supported Dr. Rath's first discovery. Read how the two courageous scientists launched their historic "Call for A Scientific Effort to Abolish Heart Disease."

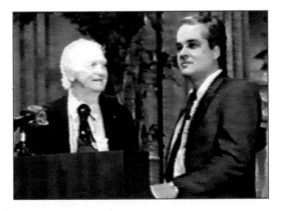

Dr. Linus Pauling and Dr. Matthias Rath at the historic press conference on July 2, 1992, calling for an international campaign to eradicate heart disease.

Developing Cellular Medicine

Now, less than ten years later, after developing the foundations of Cellular Medicine, Dr. Rath has identified many more common health conditions as primarily caused by vitamin deficiency. They include high blood pressure, heart failure, diabetic circulatory problems and many forms of cancer.

Moreover, through the relentless and uncompromising efforts led by Dr. Rath, these truths have been recognized. Small and large vitamin companies are heavily embarking in research and clinical studies to finally substantiate the broad health benefits of vitamins.

Health Food Stores as Cornerstones of a New Health Care System

In this situation, the health food stores and the natural health community, including the 150 million Americans who take vitamins on a regular basis, share a responsibility.

Now every health food store in America has the opportunity to become a cornerstone of a new health care system that focuses on the natural prevention of today's common diseases, including cardiovascular disease and cancer.

After fighting this battle for more than a decade, Dr. Rath decided to share the historic record of it with the world. The authenticity of this book leaves no doubt about who has been leading the historic breakthrough towards natural health on a worldwide scale.

"Touching the Naked Soul of Man"

Standing up as an individual scientist against one of the largest industries on earth, the pharmaceutical industry, has been a tough road. It has been a battle that reached the "naked soul" of those who fought it.

Examples of political maneuvers at the highest level of government against Dr. Rath, are boycotts, attacks on his scientific achievements and on his personal integrity in a mass media economically dependent on the pharmaceutical industry.

In one of their last conversations before his death in 1994, Linus Pauling said to Dr. Rath: "Never forget that you are fighting one of the most important battles for human health. It will be long and hard." That was an understatement. The stakes were one in a thousand for the truth of David to prevail against the economic and political power of Goliath.

By sharing this information with the people in America and other countries, Dr. Rath offers them a strong message of empowerment: You can do it too. Start taking charge of your own health now. Spread this information and help make health a human right that is available to everyone.

Setting a Personal Example

Dr. Rath's life sets an example for that path. He's the son of farmers, born and raised in southern Germany. He left the farm and studied medicine. After graduation from medical school, he conducted research in cardiovascular disease. After his first publication appeared in the *Journal of the American Heart Association,* he accepted the invitation of two-time Nobel Laureate Linus Pauling to become the first Director of Cardiovascular Research at the Linus Pauling Institute in California.

Dr. Rath's scientific achievements are a good example that young people can make some of the greatest discoveries in science. Young minds have the advantage of being uncluttered with existing dogmas.

Several times in human history the discoveries of one scientist ultimately helped to save millions of lives. When Dr. James Lind discovered that scurvy, the sailor's disease, is caused by a lack of vitamin C, 40 years passed before the knowledge was applied.

Of course, Dr. Rath does not compare himself with these historic persons. However, the medical breakthrough he led, revealing that today's most common diseases are primarily caused by vitamin deficiencies and are largely preventable, has already saved tens of thousands of lives.

The fact that it has taken him less than ten years to become widely accepted speaks for his determination.

Breakthrough

in the History of Medicine

that saved millions of lives

"New truths go trough three stages.
First they are ridiculed,
second they are violently opposed and then,
finally, they are accepted
as being self-evident."
Arthur Schopenhauer

How the Heart Started to Beat

Until the 17th century, no blood circulated in the human body. From Greek and Roman doctors to the medical students in medieval European universities, the medical profession learned that everything moving in the human body, including life itself, was driven by three spirits: the veins carried the "natural spirit" the arteries carried the "vital spirit," and the nerves carried the "animal spirit."

As long as these ancient beliefs continued, life could not be understood from a scientific or medical point of view - only from a spiritual perspective. Accordingly, for more than a thousand years little progress was made in understanding the basic function of the human body, and millions of people died as a result of this medical ignorance.

One man made the difference. In 1628, William Harvey (1578 - 1657) published *The Motion of the Heart and Blood in Animals*. In this book he published for the first time that the heart is the motor of the cardiovascular system and that blood circulation, not "vital spirits," is the motor of life. He had studied the motion of the heart in animals; he conducted strikingly simple and conclusive experiments to prove blood circulation, for example, by tying a bandage tightly around the arm until no pulse could be felt.

But above all, what made the change was the readiness of William Harvey to question the teaching of thousand year old medical dogmas and discard everything that did not hold true.

The life's work of this man terminated the medieval times in medicine.

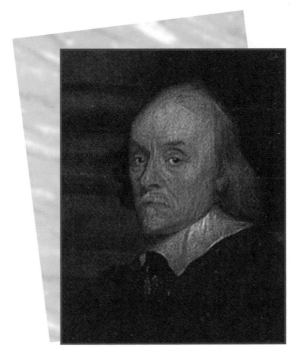

William Harvey (1578-1657)
Founder of Modern Medicine

When the Oceans Stopped Turning Red

One of the greatest threats to sailors of earlier centuries was an increased weakness of their blood vessels, bleeding, and death from massive blood loss, both inside and outside their bodies. Only a handful of sailors returned from the first efforts to circumnavigate the globe under Magellan. No one knew the cause of scurvy, this terrible disease that killed tens of thousands of sailors from the sixteenth to the eighteenth century.

Until Scottish physician James Lind (1716-1794) came along. Through a simple experiment, Lind proved that providing sufficient quantities of lime and lemon juice to the sailors could prevent bleeding and blood loss. He saved thousands of lives by finding the natural way to prevent and cure scurvy, the sailor's disease.

Today, of course, we know that the vitamin C contained in these fresh fruits is required for optimum production of collagen, connective tissue, and for optimum stability of the blood vessel walls. When Lind made his discoveries, no one cared about the exact mechanism. The main thing was that it worked.

But more surprising, it took the British Admiralty more than 40 years to put the discoveries by James Lind into practice and distribute limes to the British sailors. During those 40 years, thousands of British sailors died unnecessarily because of adherence to antiquated dogmas by the Admirality.

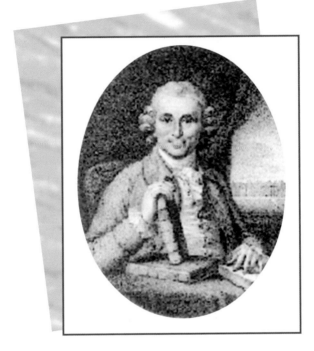

James Lind (1716–1794)
Tens of Thousands of sailors owe him their lives

Why Epidemics are no Longer a Curse of Heaven

Until the middle of the 19th century, such epidemics as plague, cholera, and smallpox were considered a curse of heaven. The sudden onset of these diseases and the lack of access to microscopes to study their real causes had kept this belief flourishing since the beginning of mankind.

Throughout the centuries hundreds of millions of people have died from epidemics, and the giant industry of incense traders, witch hunters, and other economic and philosophical interest groups thrived on the "business with epidemic diseases." Of course this business with disease would last only as long as the actual cause of epidemics remained unknown.

Everything changed with the life of the French chemist Louis Pasteur (1822-1895). By using a microscope, he was able to detect the true nature of epidemics: microorganisms. Not only did Pasteur discover the germs that caused one of the most devastating diseases of its time, rabies; he also developed the first vaccination therapy against it.

Again, one man made the difference that paved the way to the discovery of other infectious germs like tuberculosis, cholera, diphtheria and tetanus. More importantly, he enabled the development of vaccines and, later, antibiotics. Even today, hundreds of millions of people owe their lives to Louis Pasteur – mostly without knowing it.

Were the discoveries by Pasteur immediately acclaimed by the scientific community? Of course not. The French medical academy in Paris disclaimed and discredited Pasteur because he was not a doctor, but "only a chemist."

But the people of the world did not care about old dogmas. They wanted to take advantage of the new knowledge to save their own lives and those of their children. Against all initial resistance, vaccination therapy and antibiotics have led to the effective control of infectious diseases.

When Pasteur died in 1895, he was honored as a hero throughout the world for his lasting contributions to mankind.

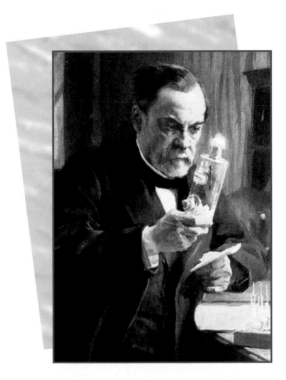

Louis Pasteur (1822-1895)
Millions of people owe him their lives

How We Learned the Origins of Diseases

The advent of the microscope also allowed a breakthrough in other areas of medicine. Until the middle of the 19th century, the causes of diseases (not only infectious diseases) were unknown. They were thought to be caused by evil spirits or bad blood. At the same time that microorganisms were discovered to cause infectious diseases and epidemics, another medical breakthrough illuminated the origin of many other diseases from within the body.

With the help of a microscope, the German physician Rudolf Virchow (1821-1902) discovered that the human body is made up of billions of cells. Furthermore, he found that diseases do not just "happen" or "possess" the body or one of its organs. He found that diseases are caused by malfunctioning cells.

These millions of malfunctioning cells eventually lead to the failure of organs, to serious health problem or disease. In 1858, Virchow published his groundbreaking *Cellular Pathology* explaining that diseases originate at the level of cells. Until this day, Virchow's *Cellular Pathology* is the foundation of pathology at the medical schools throughout the world.

Interestingly, while Virchow correctly identified the cells as the starting point for any disease, he did not identify the most frequent cause for their malfunction, a lack of bioenergy molecules essential for the optimal energy supply to each cell. The explanation is simple: vitamins and other essential carriers of cellular bioenergy were not discovered until the early decades of the 20th century – long after Virchow's death.

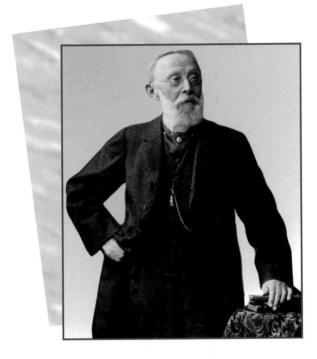

Rudolph Virchow (1821-1902)
Founder of "Cellular Pathology"

I listed these examples for good reason: they tell an invaluable story about human history, the history of medicine, how millions of people had to die because antiquated and false medical dogmas were upheld against better knowledge, how the quest for the truth carried on by individuals ultimately paid off, how these pioneers in science and humanity had to endure personal attacks, stonewalling by supporters of the old system, and other hardships.

These examples also tell the encouraging story that nothing, absolutely nothing, can stifle the truth once its time has come. I hope this message will stay with my readers throughout this book and beyond. My scientific achievements in the area of cardiovascular disease and cancer will lead to the control of today's most common diseases.

Heart attacks are the number one killer in the industrial countries today. They are followed by cancer (number two) and stroke (number three).

The natural control of these diseases during the next two decades and their reduction to a fraction of today's cases will inevitably lead to increased life expectancy. Thus, these discoveries are laying the scientific basis for realization of an old dream of mankind: longevity.

Let's look at the scope of these discoveries from another angle.

Extending the Human Body

Some of the most recent discoveries of our time that have changed human life – and were also considerable economic successes – had one thing in common: they were inventions that extended certain parts of the human body.

Thomas Edison (1847-1931). From the dawn of time human activity was confined to daylight. With the exception of torches, candles and other fire tools,

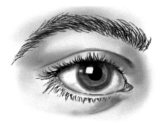

human productivity and social life were cut in half by the simple fact that human beings cannot see in the dark. The discovery of electricity, the invention of the light bulb and its mass production, changed that forever. Suddenly, **eyesight** was extended.

Alexander Graham Bell (1847-1922). Since the inception of mankind, communication between people had been confined

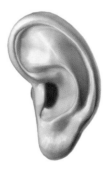

to a shouting distance. The telegraph and its precursors made first steps to change that. But it was the invention of the telephone and its network that **extended the mouth and ears** of everyone.Suddenly communication became possible from any one place to another place anywhere in the world. With this invention,another old dream of mankind had come true – communication without borders.

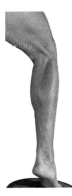

Henry Ford (1863-1947). Another ancient dream of mankind was to travel anywhere at any time. Although others invented the automobile, Henry Ford allowed this dream to come true for a majority of the population. It was he who **extended the legs** of millions and fulfilled this old dream of mankind and who was one of the first entrepreneurial benefactors.

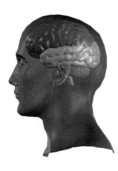

Bill Gates. (1955-present). Since the beginning of mankind, progress has been confined by the limitations of the brain to store information, do calculations, writings, information exchange and other functions. Even though computers were developed earlier, Bill Gates is credited for understanding the need for computers to serve the individual human being. He enabled millions of people to **extend their brain functions.**

But one of the greatest discoveries remained to be made: The extension of not just a single organ or body function, but of life itself – **longevity**.

This book is an account of this discovery.

The Scientific Key to Longevity

The largest of all human organs is the blood vessel system. Arteries, veins, and millions of capillaries in one body together total 60,000 miles in length, and equal the surface area of a football field. The blood vessel system has the tremendous task of providing oxygen and nutrients to literally each cell of the human body. If blood flow is impaired, millions of cells suffocate or cease to function properly because of malnutrition.

Our body is as old as our blood vessel system. This is a medical law. Thus, the earlier blood vessels harden, the shorter our lives. Vice versa, optimum health of our cardiovascular system adds years to our lives.

Maintaining the stability and proper function of the blood vessel pipeline and preventing its hardening is the first and foremost goal to extending life expectancy.

The scientific discovery that, similar to scurvy, vitamin deficiency weakens the blood vessel walls and facilitates the development of cardiovascular disease, is therefore of utmost importance for every human being. The first patented therapy for the natural prevention and reversal of cardiovascular disease is the scientific key to longevity.

This discovery, supported by progress made in other areas of vitamin research, is likely to push the average life expectancy beyond 100 years within the first half of this century.

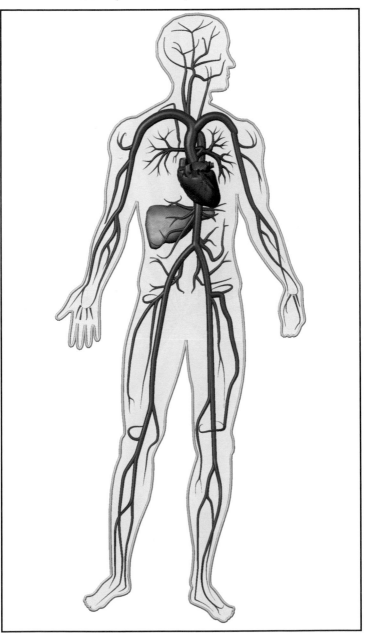

Breakthroughs in Natural Health

that will save millions of lives

"Discovery is seeing what everyone saw and thinking what no one thought."

Albert Szent-Gyoergy
Nobel Laureate, Discoverer of Vitamin C

Solving Scientific Puzzles

A scientific breakthrough rarely consists of one single observation. It is made by finding the answers to a series of questions that remained unanswered. Of particular importance are scientific breakthroughs in medicine - the sooner they are made, the fewer people who will die. Thus, medical breakthroughs can save millions of lives today and in generations to come. The solution to cardiovascular disease is no exception.

Solving scientific puzzles is like a chess game. The pictures on the opposite page illustrate that. The chess board represents the entire problem - in this case cardiovascular disease, and the question: "Why do millions of people die from heart attacks and strokes?"

The black figures represent all the fundamental unanswered questions, for example:

- Why don't animals get heart attacks, but every year heart attacks are the primary cause of death in humans?

- Why do people get infarctions in the coronary arteries of the heart (heart attacks) but no one has ever seen nose attacks, ear attacks or infarctions in the veins?

- Why do animals with high levels of cholesterol in the blood avoid heart attacks? The bear and other animals that sleep during winter (hibernators) have cholesterol levels of 600 mg/dl and higher. Why are they not extinct from an epidemic of heart attacks?

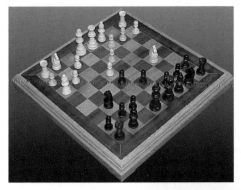

*The **cholesterol - heart disease theory** can not answer the most basic questions about cardiovascular disease:*
The black figures (unanswered questions) are still standing.

*The **scurvy - heart disease discovery** provides answers to all basic questions about cardiovascular disease: The white figures (answers) have eliminated the black ones (questions). This means:*
"Checkmate to heart disease!"

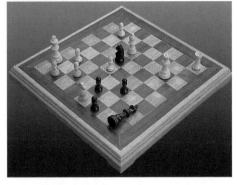

The white figures represent the answers that the scientist finds to the basic questions. The scientist leading a breakthrough gradually answers all the questions that have remained a mystery. Alternative explanations are ruled out and the problem is cornered. A breakthrough is the "Checkmate" of a scientific or medical problem.

The discovery of the scurvy/heart disease connection can answer all the questions about cardiovascular disease that were not answered by previous theories. This discovery represents the "Checkmate" to heart attacks, strokes, high blood pressure and other common diseases.

Why We Don't Get Infarctions of the Ears and Noses

Once the initial observation of the lipoprotein (a)/ vitamin C connection was made, the entire puzzle of human cardiovascular disease was solved with mathematical precision. On the following pages I will take you along the path my own mind took during this discovery process.

The blood vessel system in your body – the arteries, veins and capillaries together – measures more than 60,000 miles in length! If high cholesterol levels were the culprit, damage and clogs would occur along the entire length of the blood vessel system – we would get infarctions of the nose, ear, elbows at an equal rate. However, more than 95% of all infarctions occur in the coronary arteries of the heart - with a total length of only 10 inches!

The adjacent picture illustrates this phenomenon. The total surface area of all blood vessels in your body is about the size of a football field. Each of the squares in the picture represents an area of ten square feet. Yet the system fails again and again at the same spot – the coronary arteries. The likelihood that this is a coincidence is one in a hundred trillion – in other words: it is no coincidence. Finding the answer to this phenomenon was the second scientific step towards solving the puzzle of cardiovascular disease.

Since 95% of all clogging occurs in one organ, the heart, the answer to this question must lie in the heart itself. What sets the heart apart from all other organs in our body?

The "Plumber's Riddle"

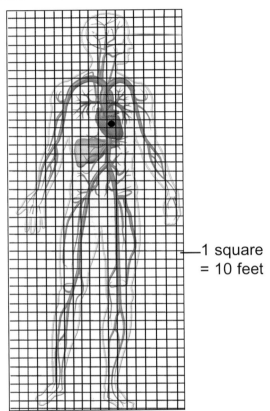

—1 square
= 10 feet

With a surface area of more than half an acre, the cardiovascular system is the largest organ in our body. Yet in 95% of the cases, clogging occurs at exactly the same spot. I gave this phenomenon the name "Plumber's Riddle" because every plumber knows that bad water quality clogs a water pipe along its entire length - not just at one spot!

E = mc² of Medicine

The heart is the only organ that constantly moves. With 100,000 heartbeats each day, the heart bears the greatest amount of mechanical stress among all organs. Particularly stressed are the walls of the coronary arteries "riding" on the surface of the heart. With each heartbeat, these arteries are squeezed flat by the muscle tension and sheer forces of the pumping heart.

After I identified the answer to this puzzle, I moved on to the next question: Why do not all people get heart attacks? If the mechanical stress from the pumping heart is such an important factor, then everyone should automatically get a heart attack from the gradual deterioration of the coronary arteries with more than 100,000 heartbeats a day or two billion squeezes of the coronary arteries over a 60-year life-cycle.

Obviously, there must be a second factor involved that determines whether we get a heart attack. This factor is the stability of the artery wall itself. But what determines this stability? The walls of the coronary arteries, just like any other blood vessels, are made up of connective tissue. The key architectural molecule of the connective tissue is collagen. Collagen has a function in the walls of the blood vessels similar to iron reinforcement rods in a skyscraper - guaranteeing stability.

Do all people have the same amount of functional collagen molecules in their arteries? Of course not. The production of collagen molecules in the body depends primarily on the supply of available vitamins and other essential nutrients like the amino acids lysine and proline. Since we human beings are unable to manufacture vitamin C or lysine in our bodies - essential nutrients in our body must come from our diet or in the form of nutritional supplements.

Why We Get Heart Attacks
and Not Nose Attacks

A   **B**

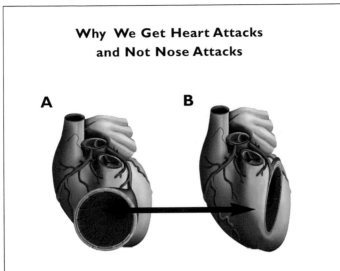

The heart beats more than 100,000 times a day. This has an immediate effect on the coronary arteries supplying blood to the heart muscle. They "ride" on top of the heart and with every pumping action of this huge muscle, these small arteries are squeezed flat.

*The above figure shows the rhythmical change in the diameter of the coronary arteries during the heart pumping cycle. During the filling phase of the heart (**A**), the heart muscle is relaxed and the coronary artery is wide. In contrast, during the pumping phase (**B**), the heart muscle is tense and the coronary artery is squeezed flat.*

This constant change occurs with every single heartbeat, about 4,000 times every hour. Imagine stepping on a garden hose 4,000 times. If the hose is new, nothing will happen. However, if the hose is weak, it will become brittle and cracks will form at precisely the spot that is constantly squeezed.

That is why we get infarctions of the heart and not of the nose or ears or eyebrows.

Thus, we have identified the second factor in our heart attack equation:

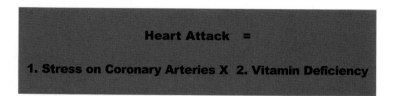

Heart Attack =

1. Stress on Coronary Arteries X 2. Vitamin Deficiency

The first factor, the pumping heart, cannot be changed. It is a constant. The heart beats, otherwise we are dead. We can only change the second factor, the amount of vitamins we take. The amount of vitamins we take is the only variable of this equation. The laws of mathematics allow the elimination of a constant. What remains is the remarkable equation:

Heart Attacks = Vitamin Deficiency

The basic puzzle of cardiovascular disease was solved with mathematical precision. No scientist, no mathematician, no health professional, no regulatory agency and, above all, no logically thinking person can dispute this fact any longer. Because of its striking similarity to Einstein's formula "$E=mc^2$" I baptized this formula the "$E=mc^2$ of Medicine."

This scientific formula is the basis for the eradication of heart disease. It will save millions of lives for generations to come.

The most frequent objection I have heard from medical professionals is that the solution to the number one health problem cannot be so simple. But it was Albert Einstein who said that the greatest scientific discoveries are so simple that they can be expressed in a way that it can be understood by everyone. The formula "$E=mc^2$ of Medicine" is no exception.

Of course there are genetic and metabolic risk factors and other mechanisms that play a role in the build-up of athero-sclerotic deposits and heart attacks. But as we shall see from the further discoveries, they are all connected to vitamin deficiency.

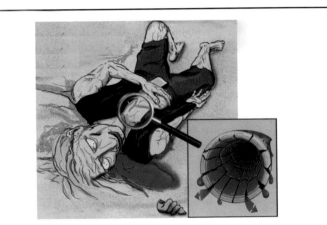

Cardiovascular disease is an early form of scurvy

Vitamin C deficiency leads to a weakening of the arteries. Centuries ago, thousands of sailors died from vitamin deficiencies at a time when vitamins were unknown.

Today, vitamins are known and available for everyone. And yet, millions of people die from cardiovascular disease and other vitamin deficiency conditions.

Why Animals Don't Get Heart Attacks - But People Do

The next puzzle I solved was "Why do animals avoid heart attacks?" The answer is: They produce their own vitamin C, sufficient for optimum collagen produc-tion and stability of their arteries. We humans cannot manufacture vitamin C and our ancestors were prone to scurvy. Threatened by extinc-tion, their bodies developed molecules to repair the artery walls weakened by vitamin deficiency.

The next discovery was identification of the most important mechanism: how our body repairs the artery walls. Among these repair molecules, one is particularly efficient - lipopro-tein(a). This molecule carries cholesterol and other fats as building blocks for new artery wall tissue, and a biological adhesive tape wrapped around it glues this molecule to the inside of the artery walls. There lipoprotein(a) binds to the most important clotting factor, fibrin, in order to stop leakage of the artery wall and early scurvy.

The next question I answered was: "Why do the deposits in the artery wall develop, and eventually clog them?" With insuffucient vitamin intake over many years, the artery wall becomes weaker, and more and more repair becomes nec-essary. Eventually the repair efforts overshoot and the deposits develop. Thus, the deposits leading to heart attacks are no longer the result of "bad luck" or a "curse of heaven." Their true nature has been revealed:

Atherosclerotic deposits are Nature's plaster cast for an artery wall weakened by vitamin deficiency.

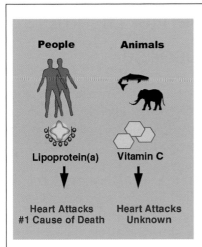

People	Animals
Lipoprotein(a)	Vitamin C
↓	↓
Heart Attacks #1 Cause of Death	Heart Attacks Unknown

Animals don't get heart attacks because they produce their own vitamin C. We humans can not manufacture vitamin C and - instead - use repair molecules to mend the artery walls.

Lipoprotein(a) molecules (yellow) enter the blood vessel wall through the cracks and crevices that form in a vitamin deficient artery wall.

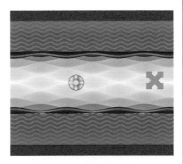

Inside the wall they bind to the clotting factor fibrin (green) and to other molecules. Over time this repair overshoots and atherosclerotic deposits form.

Atherosclerotic deposits are Nature's plaster cast for an artery wall weakend by vitamin deficiency.

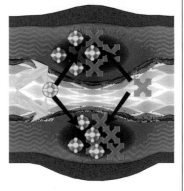

Why Most Congenital Disorders Lead to Heart Disease

One of my most amazing discoveries answers the question: why do almost all congenital diseases – in one way or another – lead to a thickening of the artery wall? The answer is logical that one wonders why no one thought of it before.

During thousands of years of the Ice Ages, half of Europe and half of the North American continent were covered with glaciers. From skeletons we know that our ancestors lived in tundra regions. The irregular structure of the bones found from these ancestors also tell us of the biggest problem for their survival: malnutrition. In areas of frozen soil there were no plants or other sources of vitamin-rich nutrition.

During the Ice Ages, epidemics of scurvy became the greatest threat to the survival of our ancestors – not just during one winter – but over hundreds of generations.

Children of Ice Age families survived these harsh conditions and reached adulthood only if they had inherited repair molecules. These repair molecules had to accomplish one task: to mend or thicken the artery walls during long periods of vitamin deficiency. Once these repair factors had appeared in one generation, they were passed on to all following generations in the genes. Today we call them "risk factors," "inherited diseases" or "family history" and we now understand why most of them cause cardiovascular disease.

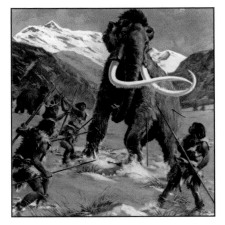

The final Ice Age lasted tens of thousands of years. The sites of Chicago, New York and other regions of North America and Europe were covered with thick ice. Malnurition-especially vitamin deficiecy-became a major cause of death.

During thousands of years of the Ice Ages, most childen died from scurvy and blood loss.

The only children to survive had inherited lipoprotein(a) or another repair molecule that thickened their artery walls during vitamin deficiencies.

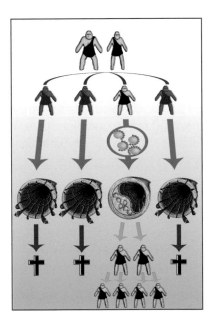

Winning the Battle Against Heart Disease

Every year twelve million people worldwide die from heart attacks and strokes, and this number is increasing. Whenever a disease expands further, it means that its true nature has not been understood.

The only country where cardiovascular disease has decreased over the last three decades is the United States. This decrease is exactly paralleled by more than a fivefold increase in the average intake of vitamins and other essential nutrients. This obvious connection, however, is disputed by interest groups that want to maintain the "business with disease."

My two scientific publications "Solution to the Puzzle of Cardiovascular Disease" and "Unified Theory of Cardiovascular Disease Leading to the Abolition of this Disease" provide the foundation of a new understanding of heart disease that ends any speculation about its true nature as a vitamin deficiency condition.

Here are the cornerstones of this new understanding:

- The stability of the blood vessel wall – not the level of cholesterol in the blood – determines the development of this disease.

- Cholesterol is a risk factor only if the blood vessel wall is already weakened by vitamin deficiency. Bears and other hibernating animals producing their own vitamin C in optimum amounts do not develop cardiovascular disease even with blood cholesterol levels of 600 mg/dl and more.

A page from the manuscript of my landmark publication
"Unified Theory of Cardiovascular Disease Leading to the Abolition of
This Disease," dated June 10, 1991.

- Cardiovascular disease is caused by a deficiency of vitamins and other essential bioenergy factors in artery wall cells responsible for the integrity and stability of the blood vessel wall.

- The atherosclerotic deposit is identified as Nature's plaster cast for an artery wall weakened by vitamin deficiency.

- We now understand why most people get infarctions of the heart and in only a few cases infarctions of other organs.

- We now know that all metabolic risk factors for cardiovascular disease known in cardiology today are associated with vitamin deficiency.

- We also know that all congenital diseases leading to cardiovascular disease are associated with and aggravated by vitamin deficiency.

- We now understand why animals don't get heart attacks but people do.

- We now know why cardiovascular disease increases dramatically after age 45.

- Above all, we now know that optimum supply of vitamins to the cells of the blood vessel walls is the key for prevention of cardiovascular disease.

The details of this medical breakthrough are clearly explained in my book, *The Heart*.

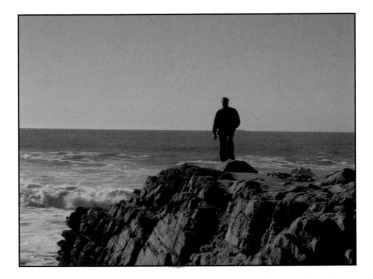

New discoveries that change the medical universe are rarely made in the laboratory. They are made in an environment that stimulates creative thinking.

By the Pacific Ocean near the small coastal town of Pescadero was my favorite location, and many of the discoveries summarized in this chapter were first conceived there.

Cellular Medicine

The next step in the series of medical breakthroughs was the most important one: The identification of vitamin deficiency and lack of cellular bioenergy as the primary cause not only of atherosclerosis but also of today's most common diseases.

The principles of Cellular Health are as follows:

1. Health and disease are determined on the level of millions of cells which compose our body and its organs.

2. Vitamins and other essential nutrients are needed for thousands of biochemical reactions in each cell. Chronic deficiency of these vitamins and other essential nutrients is the most frequent cause of malfunction of millions of body cells and the primary cause of cardiovascular and other diseases.

3. Cardiovascular diseases are the most frequent diseases because cardiovascular cells consume vitamins and other essential nutrients at a high rate due to mechanical stress on the heart and the blood vessel wall.

4. Optimum dietary supplementation of vitamins and other essential nutrients is the key to prevention and an effective treatment of cardiovascular disease, as well as other chronic health conditions.

Over the years, studies were published showing that one or another vitamin or mineral benefits patients with one or another health condition. But these were like mosaics. The complete picture was not seen until the foundation of Cellular Health and Cellular Medicine.

Never before was the deficiency of cellular energy described as the primary cause of an entire group of diseases, including high blood pressure, heart failure, diabetic circulatory problems, among others.

The application of this knowledge in daily medical practice will help millions of people and greatly reduce these diseases.

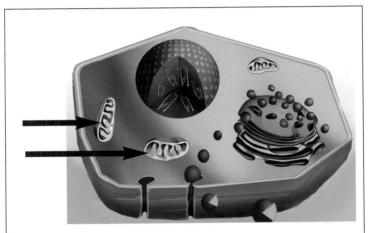

Vitamins and other essential nutrients are required as bioenegy molecules or cell fuel for the proper function of cells irrespective of the type of cell . The blue cellular power plants (mitochondriae) are the sites where vitamins are needed for cellular energy production.

My recommendation for patients with any form of cardiovascular disease: Take this book to your doctor. Start as soon as possible on a well defined vitamin program. Inform your doctor about it. Take the vitamins in addition to your prescription medication and do not discontinue or change any medication without the advice of your doctor. Above all, start soon to take advantage of this knowledge.

How it All Started

"Dr. Rath's discoveries will be considered among the most important of the 20th century"

Two-time Nobel laureate Linus Pauling (1901-1994)

How I Got Interested in Cardiovascular Research

During my last year in medical school, my father died from a heart attack and there was nothing anyone could do about it. This situation left me with the strong desire to dedicate some of my time as a medical doctor to cardiovascular research. It is the dream of every researcher to help prevent cardiovascular disease more efficiently and perhaps control this disease. Little did I know at that time that I would one day have the privilege of solving the puzzle of cardiovascular disease - thereby helping to save million of lives.

Linus Pauling told me in the early eighties that "If you want to be a good doctor you need to do research first." I followed that advice and immediately after graduation went into a research project sponsored by the German Research Foundation at the medical clinic of Hamburg University. The goal of this research project was to identify the ways by which cholesterol and other fat particles stick to the blood vessel wall. The mid-eighties were the heydays of cholesterol-lowering drugs and, accordingly, the focus of the international research community was on "bad cholesterol,"or LDL, being the main factor that causes atherosclerotic plaques, and eventually, heart attacks and strokes.

Rather than following this conventional research, I was intrigued by lipoprotein(a), a new risk factor - like "adhesive." Our own studies involving more than ten thousand research data and measurements left no doubt that in order for the "bad cholesterol" to stick inside the blood vessel wall, it needs the biological adhesive lipoprotein(a). The results established together with my colleagues were an important milestone towards understanding the nature of cardiovascular disease. We found that wherever cholesterol was deposited in the blood vessel wall there was the biological adhesive tape, apo(a). It was clear that the deposits were not dependent on the amount of cholesterol but on the amount of "adhesive" present in the body. At that point we did not know that this would be only the partial truth and that heart attacks and strokes would prove to be primarily the result of vitamin deficiencies.

These discoveries on the "sticky cholesterol" lipoprotein(a) were so new that the American Heart Association (AHA) did not accept the presentation of these data at their annual convention in 1988. They simply did not believe it. One year later the AHA invited me to give a presentation at their annual convention. At the same time the AHA accepted these findings in their official journal *Arteriosclerosis*.

Lipoprotein(a) turned out to be a a risk factor ten times greater than cholesterol. More importantly, no drugs, not even cholesterol-lowering drugs were able to lower this risk factor in the blood. But by far the most intriguing question about this new risk factor for heart attacks and strokes was the fact that it was only found in humans - rarely in other living species.

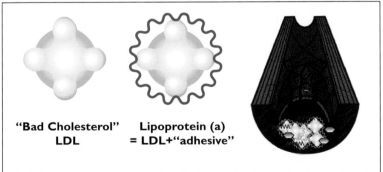

"Bad Cholesterol"
LDL

Lipoprotein (a)
= LDL+"adhesive"

"Bad Cholesterol" – or LDL – is deposited inside the vitamin deficient and weak artery wall by means of the "adhesive" lipoprotein(a).

In 1987, I made the following decisive discovery that should change medicine forever: The sticky risk factor lipoprotein(a) was only found in humans and other species that had lost the ability to manufacture their own vitamin C. Apparently, there was an inverse relationship between the lipoprotein(a) molecule and in vitamin C.deficiency. I immediately started to do experiments on vitamin C and lipoprotein(a). Later I conducted a clinical pilot study where vitamin C was shown to lower elevated lipoprotein(a) levels in patients.

Imagine the year 1987. Vitamin C was considered quackery, and no reputable medical institution was even willing to consider conducting clinical studies with vitamins. The knowledge about vitamin C as a carrier of cellular bioenergy was entirely lost in the medical education, and patentable pharmaceutical drugs were considered the only form of acceptable medicine.

I introduced my discoveries about the lipoprotein(a) / vitamin C connection to prominent researchers, among them Nobel Laureate Michael Brown from Southwestern Medical School in Dallas. They essentially rejected my discovery as a crazy idea. But I did not give up.

How I came to work with Linus Pauling

I had known Linus Pauling from the time I was a medical student. I first met him at a conference on an island in Southern Germany where young scientists had the opportunity to meet with Nobel laureates. Later I met Linus again during the Nuclear Freeze movement, and in 1983, I accompanied him on a lecture tour, where he also talked about his Nobel Peace Prize for helping to bring about the atmospheric nuclear test ban treaty. I continued to see Linus several times during the 1980's, but none of the meetings was as crucial as the one at his ranch in Big Sur in late autumn of 1989.

During the last two weeks in October that year, I made a lecture tour through the United States, presenting the work on atherosclerosis and new risk factor lipoprotein(a) that had just been published in *Arteriosclerosis*. I had been invited to present this exciting research at the Metabolic Disease branch of the National Institutes of Health in Bethesda, at the Medical School of the University of Chicago, at the Baylor College of Medicine in Houston, the Arteriosclerosis Research Department at the University of California in La Jolla and at Genentech, the famous biotech company in San Francisco. The lipoprotein(a) story was "hot news" at those ivy league research centers but any connection to vitamin metabolism was ignored.

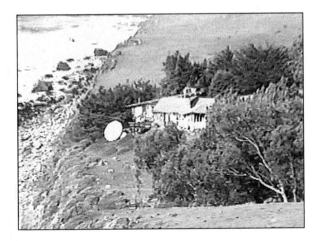

Linus Pauling's ranch on the shores of the Pacifc Ocean

The last weekend that October, I arranged a visit with Linus Pauling at his ranch in Big Sur. I had sent a copy of my publications and some supporting materials to his institute - but they never reached him. On that Saturday, I drove from San Francisco – where I had given a lecture at Genentech - to Big Sur. It was a beautiful four hour drive south along the Pacific coast. I had visited Linus at his ranch before, but this time – I knew – would be different.

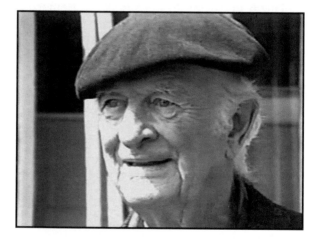

The two-time Nobel laureate at age 90
in front of his house in Big Sur

After passing the cattle gates on the small windy road from Highway 1 down to his ranch, I finally reached the wooden ranch house that Linus had chosen as his refuge for the last decades of his life. The door of his house was never locked and I entered, making my way through mountains of scientific journals that had piled up over many years along the hallway connecting the entrance with the living room. Linus was sitting in a wire chair that apparently had survived several decades. The living room looked like the epicenter of a continuous scientific whirlwind. There were books, scientific articles, and handwritten notes addressing the unsolved puzzles in physics, the atomic structure of quasi-crystals. Linus had been working for the past several months identifying these structures – using only his mind and a calculator.

Linus had not noticed me coming in. When he did, he jumped up. "Hello, Matthias, good to see you. I understand that today we are talking about your scientific work. I am glad you became a researcher." With that, he moved his chair to the balcony window and offered me the chair opposite him. I started to talk about the new risk factors lipoprotein(a) and about my discovery that this molecule only appears in humans and other species that had lost the ability to manufacture their own vitamin C. I immediately came to the point: "Linus there is an obvious connection between lipoprotein(a) and a lack of vitamin C that no one had seen before." With the waves of the Pacific Ocean smashing against the rocks below, Linus listened and asked questions. He had never heard of lipoprotein(a) before. After about an hour he stood up and said: "Well there are about a thousand papers on vitamin C each year, what is really new about this?"

It was one of these typical tests by which the eminent scientist who had seen a century in science tested the young scientist about his own convictions. I replied: "Linus, I would like to make a suggestion, I'll leave these papers here for you to read and I will stay overnight in the Ragged Point Inn. I will come back tomorrow and we can talk some more." I had passed Linus' test and he replied smiling: "Very well." I drove back to Highway 1, convinced that the next day I would know from the brightest scientist alive whether my observations are only coincidence or whether it is a principle of nature.

The Ragged Point Inn, several miles south of Linus' ranch is directly above the Pacific. I read and worked late into the night to prepare myself further for next morning's discussion. I knew that the amino acid lysine would possibly block the lipoprotein(a) fat particles from accumulating inside the artery walls. I drew figures about the combination of lysine with vitamin C modifying these lysine molecules into hydroxy-lysine, possibly preventing blood vessel deposits, heart attacks, and strokes. For California, the next morning was the beginning of another beautiful, late autumn day. For mankind, it was an historic day - the beginning of the end of the cardiovascular epidemic. When I reached Linus's ranch at nine o'clock, he was already waiting for me. He sprang from his chair and welcomed me with excitement. "I read your stuff and it is pretty interesting," he said, trying to appear controlled. However, there was no way he could hide his excitement. We talked for another three hours, during which I introduced Linus to the possible therapeutic value of vitamin C in combination with lysine, not only to prevent the deposition of this dangerous fat particle inside the artery walls but also to reverse cardiovascular diseases naturally - by releasing lipoprotein(a) from these deposits.

Linus agreed, but he seemed more fascinated by the evolutionary connection, the loss of vitamin C production in the ancestor of man and the sudden appearance of lipoprotein (a) a few hundred thousand years ago. "Isn't it amazing that this particle popped up in such a short time during evolution?" he asked. I realized that Linus looked at scientific problems in a fundamentally different way than all the other scientists. His intellect covered millions of years in evolution as easily as the atomic structure of atoms no one had ever seen.

I felt pretty proud of having excited this scientific giant with my discoveries. This Sunday morning ended in small talk, with

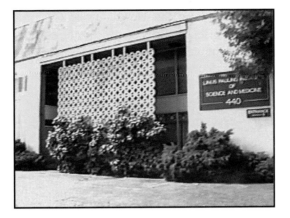

The Linus Pauling Institute on 440 Page Mill Road in Palo Alto in 1990. The building was torn down in 1998.

Linus asking me about continuing my research in California and even explaining to me the size of his property and the possibility to build one or two more houses on that property. I did not immediately understand the reason why he broached this matter until much later. He was a scientist buried alive with his life's work on vitamins. He had just met with a young scientist with whom he not only shared his views for a better world, but also a common scientific drive to get the health benefits for vitamins accepted on a worldwide scale.

When we parted, Linus said: "Matthias, this is a very important discovery. But I don't think I should get more involved in this than just talking to you." Apparently, he felt he had not contributed to this discovery and that he should rather continue his current research in physics. This was all I needed to hear, a confirmation of my discovery as a principle of Nature by the two-time Nobel laureate. Elated, I jumped in my rental car and drove the eight hours south to San Diego. The next day I would have a presentation at the cardiovascular research department of the University of California at La Jolla. But this was today - my day! I remember honking at cows, seals and just about any other creature that crossed my way south that sunny October afternoon.

Four days later I was back in Berlin, Germany, and two days afterwards I received a letter from Linus Pauling. He had given up his professed indifference and given way to open enthusiasm. He proposed writing a scientific publication for the *Proceedings of the National Academy of Science* about the connection between lipoprotein(a) and vitamin C deficiency. More importantly, he invited me to join his institute, start a cardiovascular research group, and become his personal collaborator.

Of course, Linus did not escape the dreadful state of affairs at his institute at that time. In his letter I found the sentence, "I even think we have an ultracentrifuge at the institute." The availability of an ultracentrifuge, of course, was just about the minimum equipment for any reputable research laboratory. I knew the research possibilities at The Pauling Institute would be very limited.

I pondered this gracious invitation for a night, and the next day I called Linus. I thanked him for the invitation but declined it. I had decided to continue this research project at the Baylor College of Medicine in Houston, a major medical institution. My explanation to Linus was straightforward: "Linus, if I come to work with you on vitamin C, it is like all Catholics moving to the Vatican. I want to take vitamin research into established medicine in order to accelerate its acceptance for mainstream medicine." After a long pause, Linus responded, "Very well."

Little did I know that this decision would not last more than six weeks. After a short interlude at the Baylor College of

Medicine in January 1990, my fascination with collaborating with the two-time Nobel Laureate was overwhelming. I packed my suitcases and moved from Houston to Palo Alto.

Working at the Linus Pauling Institute

I remember the day in early 1990 when I drove into Palo Alto I was full of ideas and plans to confirm this principle of nature at the experimental level at the Pauling Institute.

At 440 Page Mill Road, I stopped my car. This was the Linus Pauling Institute where I had met with Linus during my student days. This time it was different. Here would be my new work place and one of the greatest rides in the history of medical science was waiting for me. I was excited.

Besides Linus, no one knew about the forthcoming scientific earthquake and the sequence of explosions that would detonate at this rather uneventful institute. In order to cover the true nature of this discovery and to protect it from curious colleagues, Linus and I agreed on code language about this project. Even the lecture I had given in early January to the employees of the Pauling Institute had been on the lipoprotein(a) work alone - without mentioning any connection to vitamin C which, of course, was the truly exciting part of it.

The next morning Linus and I met with the President of the Linus Pauling Institute. Linus addressed him directly: "I want everyone at the institute to know that Matthias is my personal protégé." Later I realized that the two-time Nobel Laureate had made this statement not only based on his friendship and common scientific interests with me but also because he was aware that his institute had become a mine field.

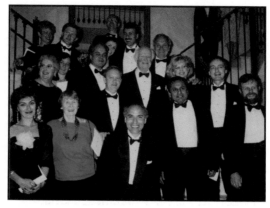

Colleagues from the Linus Pauling Institute at the Nobel laureate's 90th birthday in 1991. Several of them later joined Dr. Rath's research firm and still work with him. Among them Dr. Alexandra Niedzwiecki (right of Linus Pauling) and Martha Best (same row far left). At the center left of the bottom row is Dorothy Munro, Linus Pauling's secretary for two decades.

For two decades the Pauling Institute had been in existence but had lost its profile as a vitamin research institute. Only one out of ten researchers even worked on vitamin C, and millions of dollars in donations from around the world were wasted for research not even remotely related to documenting the health benefits of vitamins. Linus' last book, *How To Live Longer and Feel Better,* listed two hundred supporting references but few came from his own institute! Clearly, the Nobel Laureate had entrusted his institute to the hands of people who were averse to leading the battle for the acceptance of vitamins for health! Tens of thousands of readers of Linus Pauling's books connected his name with ongoing vitamin research, but the administration of his institute was ashamed of controversies and of taking up the good fight for natural health.

In this situation, Linus at age 90 had obviously realized that this could be his last opportunity to find a young and enthusiastic researcher to carry on his life's work. However, his announcement that I was his protégé could not have been more threatening to the existing leadership of the Linus Pauling Institute. And I should soon feel the consequences. Instead of getting a decent work place with a desk and chair, I was allocated the corner seat in the windowless storage area of the Pauling Institute. My request to the Institute's administration for a research assistant who could help in laboratory was met with the argument that the Institute did not have money.

Not willing to give up, I trained the janitor to run the electropheresis experiments in the laboratory so I could concentrate on elaborating the details of this medical breakthrough. Weeks, perhaps months, were lost and it was not until a year later that I finally got a qualified research assistant.

Key Experiments for the Medical Breakthrough

I had already made the principal discovery of the vitamin C deficiency – lipoprotein(a) connection back in 1987. Now the door was wide open to scientific proof. I set up a study with guinea pigs, an animal that shares the same genetic defect as human beings. These animals cannot produce their own vitamin C. The experiment was straightforward. My theory was that guinea pigs develop atherosclerotic deposits once they are put on a vitamin C deficient diet. Moreover, by analyzing the deposit in the artery walls we would find the sticky lipoprotein(a) fat molecules.

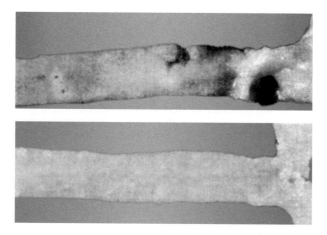

Top: Guinea pigs receiving too little vitamin C in the diet develop cardiovascular disease.
Bottom: Guinea pigs receiving optimum vitamin C have clean arteries.

The significance of this experiment for the lives and health of millions of people could not be underestimated. This experiment would conclude that a similar mechanism takes place in the human body. The lack of vitamin C would weaken the blood vessel walls, and subsequently lipoprotein(a), cholesterol and other risk factors in the blood would be deposited inside the artery walls to mend them. That would prove the fatty deposits in the arteries are no longer a coincidence but that cardiovascular diseases develop as an inevitable response of the body to repair the blood vessel walls weakened by vitamin deficiency.

This key experiment was carried out over five weeks, one of the longest five weeks in my life. Of course, animal experiments must be kept to an absolute minimum, but since this experiment would impact the health and lives of millions of people, it had been approved by the animal care committee of the Institute. I still remember the day the experiment was over, and I looked at the artery walls of the guinea pigs under the microscope. The guinea pigs receiving vitamin C comparable to the human RDA had developed the same deposits in the artery walls that caused heart attacks and strokes. Those animals that had received the equivalent of two teaspoons of vitamin C per day compared to human body weight had maintained clean arteries. Most importantly, this striking difference was not obtained by *adding* cholesterol or fat to the diet but by *omitting* one single factor from the diet - Vitamin C.

That day I felt like Columbus must have felt at the first sight of land in 1492 - after years of struggle and overcoming adversities. I went to Dorothy Munroe, Linus Pauling's secretary and asked where I could reach Linus to share the exciting news with him. She noticed my excitement and said: "Go right in, he is in his office." I didn't even close the door behind me and shouted: "Linus, you've got to come and see this!"

He had been dictating letters and correspondence in his typical posture, half lying in his chair with his feet on the desk. His black beret was drawn deep over his eyes, in order to dim the neon light of his office. He literally jumped up, adjusted his beret and walked with me to the room where the guinea pig arteries were under the microscope. The results left no doubt: Optimal amount of vitamin C was the solution to the cardiovascular epidemic.

After looking through the microscope for a few minutes, Linus rose, turned around and beamed at me: "I am happy as a clam." He took me by the arm and we went to his office to discuss the next steps, as well as the implications for human health.

That evening, when I drove home, I knew that medicine would never again be the same. Thoughts were appearing like flashes in my mind and a breathtaking perspective was opening up. I saw people around the world embracing this discovery and researchers tuning in to further confirm them at all levels. I imagined the morning news opening up with the headline: "Heart Disease Close to Eradication." I could see a new research institute rising into the sky. How could I know that the fight for acceptance of this simple truth had just began and that years of fierce battles lay ahead of me.

Irritation Everywhere

The first reactions to this medical breakthrough, the publications and the lipoprotein(a)/ vitamin C deficiency connection, were sheer irritation. Imagine the times in 1991. The world was in full swing on the cholesterol/heart disease connection. Every major pharmaceutical company had invested multi-million dollar advertising budgets for new cholesterol-lowering drugs with the hope of capitalizing on the illusion of combating heart disease by lowering cholesterol. Only the top one percent of the research community had even heard about lipoprotein(a) and accepted that it is a ten times greater risk factor for heart disease than cholesterol.

Now, along comes a young German scientist publishing the outrageous conclusion that this prominent risk factor, lipoprotein(a), can be successfully neutralized by optimum intake of vitamin C. Moreover, with a flash of his scientific mind, he shook almost every scientific explanation for heart disease that had ever existed. To top it off, for these bold conclusions, he recieved the support of Linus Pauling, the only scientist ever to receive two unshared Nobel Prizes.

Only during the times of Harvey, Pasteur, and a few others, had the medical world been as challenged as it was during the years 1990-91.

Both Linus and I were fully aware of the significance of these discoveries. Before one of the inevitable business negotiations, Linus said: "I can't give you any specific advice. You have to use your own judgment. But no matter what happens, never forget that your discovery is one of the most important discoveries in medicine ever." Even more surprising was the fact that a public debate about this breakthrough essentially did not take place. Only later would I understand why.

Instead, the reactions at this time were a mixture of astonishment, irritation, and desperate efforts to contain the wildfire started by this medical breakthrough. As we shall see throughout this book, the prevailing reactions were erratic efforts to contain the spread of this discovery, combined with economic greed of galactic proportions.

Of course, it was clear that neither the pharmaceutical industry nor any of the scientists or doctors on their payroll would publicly contradict the logic of this medical breakthrough. Ever since James Lind showed that lime and lemon juice prevent scurvy, it was clear that vitamin C would stabilize the artery wall and also protect it against the damages associated with cardiovascular disease. This logic had the multi-billion dollar pharmaceutical "strato-dwellers" shaking in their boots.

Every strategic move they planned during those years was only viable under one condition: it would have to guarantee that the information about this medical breakthrough would be contained and no public education about the possibility of eradicating heart disease with vitamins could be spread. Since my discovery was a global threat to the "Business with Disease," the pharmaceutical companies reacted in a global way.

In later chapters of this book, I will describe in detail how the pharmaceutical industry formed two cartels; one became infamous as the so-called "vitamin cartel." This global cartel was an effort by the world's leading manufacturers of vitamin raw materials to suck the life from this medical breakthrough through criminal price-fixing practices. The other became known as the "Pharma-Cartel," an effort by the pharmaceutical industry to limit health claims and the dissemination of any preventive and therapeutic health information on vitamins and other non-patentable natural therapies. The common denominator of these two cartels was that neither roquired the release of the medical breakthrough about the role of vitamins in prevention of heart disease, information that hundreds of millions of people were waiting for because it could have saved or prolonged their lives.

As an expression of the erratic behavior of the leading scientists and pharmaceutical companies, I would like to share some of the moments during that year that tell more than any historic analysis ever could.

"Cholesterol-Popes" and Shattered Dogmas

In 1985, Goldstein and Brown, two researchers from the University of Texas, received the Nobel Prize for discovering a pathway by which cholesterol enters the cells. While this discovery was significant, the Nobel Prize these two gentlemen received was advertised by the drug companies that manufactured cholesterol-lowering drugs as the "final proof" for their questionable theory that cholesterol caused heart disease. Of course, these two researchers were not independent; they had rather lucrative consulting arrangements with pharmaceutical companies, among them Genentech Inc. in South San Francisco.

Our first paper about the lipoprotein(a)/ vitamin C connection had just been published in the *National Academy of Sciences*, in May 1990. Shortly thereafter there was a meeting of scientific advisors for Genentech, in which Goldstein and Brown participated. The two gentlemen had not even been seated when they started to ask everyone in the room whether they had read the Rath/ Pauling paper on lipopro-tein(a) and vitamin C. For the two scientific gurus who had been the architects of the Babylonian Tower of the choles-terol/ heart disease connection, this very tower had just been shaken by an earthquake of a 10.0 magnitude.

Linus and I had great fun thinking about the event at which one of us would first detonate the bomb in person. I had a stand-ing invitation to an arteriosclerosis meeting in Venice, Italy, in August 1990. Nearly the entire cream of medical researchers and scientific opinion leaders in the area of cholesterol and heart disease were present. Among them were Daniel Steinberg from the University of California in La Jolla and Toni Gotto, the former president of the American Heart Association, from the Baylor College of Medicine in Houston, Texas.

My presentation was on the role of certain antioxidants in the prevention of cardiovascular disease. At the end of this talk I mentioned in a few sentences the discovery about lipopro-tein(a), vitamin C deficiency and heart disease. During the lunch hour, I distributed copies of the publication from the *Proceedings of the National Academy of Sciences*. From that moment on the conference was not the same. The mood become funereal and Toni Gotto summarized the new situa-tion for the scientists present in the following way: "If Rath and Pauling are correct, then everything is different anyway." Of course we were correct! In hindsight, the former president of the American Heart Association may have regretted that statement. But at the time it was a genuine expression that the medical universe had just been redesigned.

Even within the Linus Pauling Institute, the irritation about this medical breakthrough was noticeable. Many noticed that Linus Pauling was supporting these far-reaching conclusions. Yet, for the researchers and the leadership of the Institute at that time, bold conclusions like the solution to the puzzle of cardio-vascular disease were unheard of. I remember that some of the researchers from other groups wanted to join me in the quest to eradicate heart disease. They were held back by their colleagues who stated that these publications were just too bold. "If you work with Dr. Rath, you will ruin your career." Of course, today we know that none of that was true, and those who joined me in this quest to eradicate heart disease have had the ride of their lives.

One of the most remarkable events surrounded the publication of our scientific papers in the *Proceedings of the National Academy of Sciences*. This scientific journal is unique because it is a rather exclusive circle of authors who are allowed to publish there. Members of the Academy may contribute a certain number of papers each year. They themselves are the reviewers for publications to be submitted. There was an unspoken arrangement between Linus and me that I would write the papers and he would submit them for publication in this prestigious journal.

The first two papers were published without any major obstacles. The problems started with the third. For this ground-breaking publication I had suggested the title, "Solution to the Puzzle of Human Cardiovascular Disease: Its Primary Cause is Ascorbate Deficiency Leading to a Deposition of Lipoprotein(a) and Fibrin/ Fibrinogen in the Vascular Wall." Linus Pauling submitted this publication to the Academy of Science. The editor-in-chief replied that he would publish it if we would agree to some minor changes. We did. However, the same editor suddenly changed his mind. Against all rules of the National Academy, he decided to have the manuscript submitted by Linus Pauling "reviewed" by anonymous colleagues. These scientists who have remained in the dark until today rejected the publication of this landmark paper with the argument: "Since there is no puzzle of cardiovascular disease, there can be no solution to this puzzle." What a remarkable statement!

I remember talking with Linus about this open act of censorship. We agreed that we should not allow ourselves to be drawn on to the chessboard of special interest groups and members of the Academy of Sciences who served those interests.

We immediately decided to publish this landmark publication in the Canadian *Journal of Orthomolecular Medicine*. I could not resist adding in the foreword the quotation from a letter from Kepler to Galilei: "My dear Kepler, what do you say of the leading philosophers here to whom I have offered a thousand times of my own accord to show my studies, but who, with the lazy obstinacy of a serpent who has eaten his fill, have never consented to look at the planets, or moon, or telescope? Verily, just as serpents close their ears, so do men close their eyes to the light of truth."

I also wrote a short introduction to this publication, detailing the censorship by the National Academy. I wanted everyone who would hold this historic publication to know how tough it was to get the truth out. Never should it be forgotten that there are interest groups so powerful that they can block publication of the scientific truth, a truth that was so important it could have saved the lives of millions of people in the meantime.

I remember talking with Linus about this censorship, I said, "One day those people responsible for the rejection of this publication will be tracked down by scientific historians. I would not want to be in their shoes. They share the responsibility for unnecessary suffering and the premature deaths of thousands, perhaps millions, of people." Linus agreed.

During those months, neither Linus nor I ever doubted that we were writing history. Our only question was how long it would take until the whole world would know and benefit from this medical breakthrough.

In the next chapter of this book, I shall summarize the milestones of this process over the last ten years. In subsequent chapters, I shall focus on overcoming the obstacles placed in my way to accomplishing this global perception change in the area of natural health.

Milestones

of the Medical Breakthrough

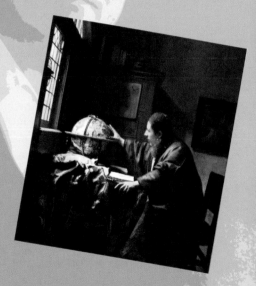

"My dear Kepler, what do you say of the leading philosophers here
to whom I have offered a thousand times of my own accord
to show my studies, but who, with the lazy obstinacy of a serpent
who has eaten his fill, have never consented
to look at the planets, or moon, or telescope?"

*Galileo Galilei in a letter to Johannes Kepler, who had discovered
that the earth circles the sun (1630 A.D.)*

Scientific Earthquake

To fully comprehend the significance of this medical break-through for worldwide human health, we need only go back a decade. When I came to America in late 1989 with the discovery that would eventually eliminate heart disease as the number one cause of death, vitamins were by no means accepted. To the contrary, they were ridiculed by the medical profession and considered a commodity by most people. The health benefits of vitamins in the prevention of cardiovascular disease and most other common diseases were neither scientifically established nor known to the public.

Of course, that was no coincidence. For more than a century, the pharmaceutical industry had systematically worked to discredit vitamins and other non-patentable therapies in order to establish their global market of patented prescription drugs. They had infiltrated not only the medical schools, but also regulatory agencies like the Food and Drug Administration (FDA) to eliminate competition from medical use of vitamins and other natural health therapies.

Vitamin products could not be sold with any reasonable health information associated with them. A health food manufacturer who ignored these strict laws did so at his own risk. Spreading health information associated with multivitamin products was considered a criminal act because - in the eyes of the law - this constituted the "criminal act" of selling an unlicensed drug.

Of course, these laws had not been made in the interests of hundreds of millions of Americans and people around the world but to serve the interest groups that had built up the pharmaceutical industry as an investment. To maintain their grip on the lawmakers, the pharmaceutical companies hired an army of lobbyists and spent billions of dollars for political "donations." In fact, the number of lobbyists in Washington surpassed the legal PR efforts of any other industry. For every Senator and Representative in Congress, two lobbyists paid by the pharmaceutical industry worked tirelessly around the clock to influence legislation according to the specifications of the drug companies.

The health food stores and the manufacturers of vitamin and natural health products had largely surrendered. No vitamin company would put out a product showing information about any life-saving health benefits of vitamins because they risked not only having to pull back the product but also faced penalties under the existing laws. Worse, since you could not use any health information relating to vitamins, vitamin companies spent insignificant amounts of money to document the health benefits of vitamins and other natural health products through research or clinical studies.

The 20th century will be known as the "Dark Ages of Medicine." Influenced by the pharmaceutical industry, mankind's knowledge about the life-saving health benefits of vitamins, minerals, amino acids, and other basic components of the metabolism of every cell in our body had been censored, ostracized, discredited, and even criminalized.

As a direct result, hundreds of millions of people worldwide died from health problems that are not diseases; they are the result of vitamin deficiencies, and therefore preventable. How could these millions of people know? How could they know if patients and doctors alike were systematically disoriented and threatened by global media campaigns organized by the PR firms of the pharmaceutical companies to discredit the health benefits of vitamins and spread lies about totally unproven health risks?

That was the state of affairs when I came to America with the discovery that heart disease could eventually be eradicated forever by simple knowledge about the benefits of vitamins and other essential nutrients. With this background, we also begin to appreciate the accomplishments over the last decades and the milestones achieved on this way. They will be summarized on the following pages.

When writing this report, I do not, by any means, want to leave the impression that without Dr. Rath we would still live in the Medieval Times of Medicine, as we found them at the end of the 1980's. To the contrary, many have contributed to implementing the changes towards liberating human health that have occurred over the last ten years.

But the fact remains that without my discoveries about vitamins and cardiovascular health, without the foundation of cellular medicine, and without the determination to defend all these against the powerful interests of the pharmaceutical industry, few, if any, of the following changes in medicine and improvements in global health would have happened:

- Vitamins and other essential nutrients have become part of established medicine. One of three doctors in America and two of three in Europe are already using vitamins and other natural health remedies in their daily practices. Ten years ago not even one out of ten doctors used natural therapies.

- In the year 2001, more than 80% of all medical schools in the United States have integrated courses on nutritional medicine, among them Harvard, Stanford, Johns Hopkins and Tufts. Before the publication of my discoveries ten years ago, fewer than five percent of the medical institutions offered such courses.

The Natural Health Revolution
Between 1990 and 2000

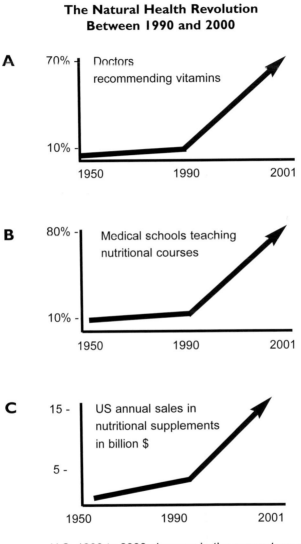

U.S. 1990 to 2000 changes in the percentage of:
A. Doctors recommending vitamins
B. Medical schools teaching nutritional courses
C. Annual sales in nutritional supplements

- In 1994, the National Institutes of Health in Bethesda, Maryland, established an Office of Alternative Medicine. Among other things, this department provides government grants for vitamin studies nationwide. Nothing like that had ever happened before in the century old history of this institution.

- Over the last ten years, the U.S. vitamin market more than doubled, from less than $5 billion in annual sales to $18 billion. In Europe, the percentage of people regularly taking vitamins increased during that time from less than five percent to more than 20 percent.

- The public perception of vitamins has changed dramatically. These natural compounds formerly regarded as commodities without clear health benefits, vitamins have become a sales pitch for many consumer products, from soaps to shampoos.

- Around the world, millions of people who had been taking vitamins without knowing the health benefits of the products are now making informed decisions. They can select multivitamin programs that address their individual needs.

In summary, during the last ten years of the 20th century, one of the greatest revolutions occurred in medicine and health care. There may still be some diehard skeptics out there who think these statistical facts are simply coincidence. These are probably the people who also believe in Santa Claus.

The fact remains that driven by scientific breakthroughs in the area of natural health, mankind was able to rip open the "iron curtain" obfuscating the health benefits of vitamins.

This silent revolution in medicine and health care that has

been taking place over the last decade has already saved millions of lives.

In the next section of my book, I will share the milestones that have been achieved during this decade, allowing this process to go forward.

The Milestones

MILESTONE:

Scientific Breakthrough

The first milestone was the discovery of the lipoprotein(a)/ vitamin C deficiency connection outlined in the earlier chapters of this book. In essence, this one molecule, lipoprotein (a), triggered my scientific interest and led to all subsequent events. By some good fortune, I had known Linus Pauling and his work on vitamin C even before I knew lipoprotein(a), and years before I was privileged to discover the close association between these two molecules.

An important part of this milestone was also the fact that Linus Pauling put his reputation as a two-time Nobel laureate behind my discovery and offered me the opportunity to continue working on this important discovery at his institute. Without Linus Pauling, my discoveries would not have received the attention and the initial push that are so important for every major change in history.

In one of our last conversations before his death in August 1994, Linus and I talked about how history would see his role in relation to vitamins and natural health. I said: "Linus, you will be credited for three things: First, to have held up the banner of health benefits of vitamins for 20 years, during which time vitamins had been demonized by the pharmaceutical industry. Second, for having invited me to join you at your institute, based on my discoveries in the area of cardiovascular health and vitamins. Third, for having given this discovery your personal support and your personal heritage to mankind in the field of human health." Linus agreed.

Early on he had seen that the the vitamin C deficiency/ scurvy/ heart disease connection would eventually integrate with his 20-year struggle for recognition of vitamins and his interests in the area of vitamin C and the common cold and vitamin C and cancer.

MILESTONE:

Informing the Medical Community

The next milestone was the vigorous effort to spread this medical breakthrough to the medical and scientific communities.

Why the Chief Cardiologist at Harvard Had to Go

I recall sending copies of my papers to the leading scientists and doctors in the field of cardiovascular research. While all of them understood it and knew that I was right, only one dared to answer in a constructive manner. Valentin Fuster, then head of cardiology at Harvard Medical School, wrote to me: "You might be quite correct in the prediction of the health benefits of vitamins." This letter also announced his own interest in this field.

The fact that I published the letter of Dr. Fuster as a first indication of support from medical opinion leaders did not help his career. He was soon ousted from his position at Harvard Medical School for political reasons.

Dr. Fuster's research has become a "silent support" of the cardiovascular disease mechanisms described in my papers - without openly referring to the benefits of vitamins. For example, he is supporting the new definition of the deposits in the artery wall as a "plaster cast" for a weakened artery wall. However, despite knowing better, he avoids addressing the most important question of all: What is the primary cause of weak arteries? Everyone knows it anyway: Vitamin deficiency.

Amazingly, in the meantime Dr. Fuster has written a two-volume manual on atherosclerosis, a standard for the American Heart Association and for generations of doctors interested in this field. With over 1600 pages, the work never

---

HARVARD MEDICAL SCHOOL —— MASSACHUSETTS GENERAL HOSPITAL

VALENTIN FUSTER, M.D., Ph.D.
Mallinckrodt Professor
of Medicine

Chief, Cardiac Unit
32 Fruit Street
Bulfinch Bldg., Room 105
Boston, MA 02114
Tel. 617-726-2887
Fax 617-726-7419

July 6, 1992

Matthias Rath, M.D.
Linus Pauling Institute of Science and Medicine
440 Page Mill Road
Palo Alto, CA 94306-2025

Dear Dr. Rath:

Unfortunately your letter a few months ago was misfiled and I found it just yesterday.

I just read your article written with Dr. Pauling on the role of ascorbic acid deficiency in vascular disease. It is an excellent article which points out the many roles of Vitamin C in the regulation of vascular processes. You may be interested to know that our own group is getting involved in this line of research. You may be quite correct in your predictions of the importance of ascorbate.

Thank you very much again for your confidence in writing to me. I wish you the best.

Sincerely,

Valentin Fuster, M.D., Ph.D.

VF/aw

mentioned vitamin C once. I can only conclude that the peer pressure from the medical establishment and those who control the "business with disease" does not allow a scientist - who knows the truth - to say it.

You, the readers of this book, you, the people, and you, the patients, must come to grips that no one will change that deplorable state of affairs – except you. This book is written to support everyone who realizes that the "business with disease" – with all its mechanisms for suppressing the truth – must be stopped as a precondition to eradicating cardio-vascular diseases.

I believe that if we continue to advocate the health benefits of vitamins in a compelling way, the leading institutions have to follow. Sooner or later, scientists and medical opinion leaders will join the vitamin research community.

Calling Upon the World's Cardiologists

to Join in the Eradication of Heart Disease

Informing the world's leading cardiologists firsthand that the disease they specialize in can be eradicated was another milestone in this historic process.

Another event I recall is distributing copies of all my scientific publications at the annual convention of the American Heart Association in November 1991 in Anaheim, California. There was a special session on lipoprotein(a), the particle that by that time had attracted the world's leading researchers of cardiovascular disease to one conference room at the Anaheim Hilton Hotel. We had prepared a set of the publications documenting how this molecule leads the way to eradicating cardiovascular disease.

My colleague, Dr. Niedzwiecki, placed a folder with these scientific publications on each chair in that room. None of the scientists and doctors could miss it. At the podium some speakers gave lectures about the fiftieth malicious property of the lipoprotein(a) molecule, but scarcely anyone was listening. They were all reading with astonishment that it is precisely this molecule that answered the puzzle of cardio-vascular disease.

To fully appreciate the impact of this event, you have to imagine yourself as one of 15,000 privileged to be invited to this most important annual event for cardiologists. Only a select group of cardiologists has the opportunity to attend these conferences. The conference catalogue was more than 100 pages thick, listing several hundred lectures and more than 1000 posters, just about every detail of cardiovascular disease. Cardiovascular disease – so it must have appeared to the senior researchers and the young cardiologists alike – was a huge mystery with many facets at the levels of organs, cells and molecules; in fact so complicated that the riddle could never be solved.

And here were the publications by Dr. Rath, the physician and scientist, whom they all knew from his earlier publica-tions on lipoprotein(a), proudly and boldly announcing the solution to the entire cardiovascular problem. Even more amazing, the solution he offered was not associated with a new surgical technique, a new device, or a pharmaceutical drug artificially developed in a drug company's reagent tube. The solution he offered was the optimum use of one of the most ancient, widespread and affordable substances of all – vitamin C. Put yourselves in the shoes of the researchers and scientists. You are left in disbelief and denial. You prob-ably would have said: "It can't be that the solution to the most widespread disease of our time is so simple!" But it is.

Interestingly, this simplicity became the greatest obstacle for doctors and scientists to accept.

Many more stories about stunned doctors and irritated medical institutions could be told. But that is not the purpose of this book. The message is this: We have done everything we could to spread this breakthrough among the medical community. We considered it our responsibility to inform the international research and cardiology community about this breakthrough, so that they could never say: "We did not know."

MILESTONE:

The First Patented Therapy for the Natural Reversal of Cardiovascular Disease

The next milestone was the application for patents for this medical breakthrough. We knew early on that the only way it could ultimately be brought to millions of people would be to develop products based on this discovery to prevent and treat cardiovascular diseases. The first patent applications were filed in early 1990, and it took four years of communication and further substantiation before the Patent Office finally approved the health claims on the use of vitamin C, lysine and other essential nutrients for the prevention and therapy of cardiovascular disease.

For any patent process, the filing date of the application is the critical date. The filing of our first patents in early 1990 enabled us to enter into talks with pharmaceutical companies without fear of their seizing the discovery other than through a licensing agreement that essentially would preserve the independent nature of this discovery and protect it from the manipulations of any drug company. This was important because we needed to insure that no matter what happened, these patents would never fall into the hands of the wrong people and buried out fear of competition with their pharmaceutical drugs.

Subsequently, several more patents were issued, but the initial decision to go this way and patent nature in order to improve the health of mankind remains a milestone of this process.

MILESTONE:

Unmasking the Drug Companies'

"Business with Disease"

After filing the patents, we contacted several pharmaceutical companies to inquire about their willingness to use their financial and marketing power to disseminate this medical breakthrough on a global level. In order to improve our negotiating position, Linus Pauling and I incorporated a small company, Therapy 2000. At age 91, he would give the name recognition - I would do the work.

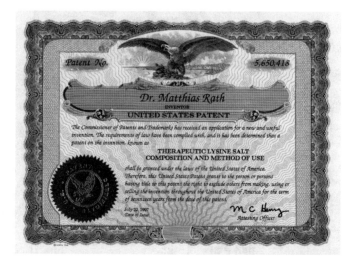

The latest in a series of patents issued by the US patent office for the natural prevention and reversal of cardiovascular disease.

In order to move forward, I hired a consultant well established in the biotech community, Dr. Alexander Cross, former vice president of Syntex, in Silicon Valley. Alex Cross was well connected to pharmaceutical companies both in the United States and in Europe. He contacted and personally visited more than a dozen of those companies to stimulate interest for the patents.

All his efforts ended in deadlock. None of the pharmaceutical companies contacted was even willing to consider a product or pharmaceutical drug based on this technology. All of them were heavily involved with cholesterol-lowering drugs and feared that research based on stabilizing the artery wall would endanger and ultimately destroy the marketing potential of cholesterol-lowering drugs for the prevention of cardiovascular disease.

I visited several companies, including Hoffmann-LaRoche, trying to persuade them to market this medical breakthrough for the benefit of themselves - and of mankind. But they were only interested in their own benefit. The dreadful chapter about Hoffmann-LaRoche will be covered later in this book when I write about the origin of the illegal price-fixing "vitamin cartel."

Schering Pharmaceuticals - "The Pill" and the

"Business with Disease"

Another remarkable chapter in this effort to find global pharmaceutical partners was my contact with Schering Pharmaceuticals. In the summer of 1999, I paid a visit to the Schering Company Headquarters in Berlin. After a brief introduction to the CEO, Mr. DeVito, I met with Dr. Rubanyi, the head of cardiovascular research of this pharmaceutical multinational and other scientists.

One reason I believed that Schering would be interested in promoting the breakthrough in vitamins and cardiovascular health was the fact that Schering is one of the world's leading producers of oral contraceptives ("The Pill"). One of the greatest health problems associated with long-term use of oral contraceptives is the severalfold increase in the risk of cardiovascular diseases. Moreover, a number of studies documented that hormonal contraceptives decrease the body's reserves of vitamin C.

One and one makes two and it was obvious to me that Schering's best-selling product, "The Pill", causes early scurvy in millions of women, weakening the artery walls and leading to heart attacks and strokes. My discoveries enabled Schering to finally address one of the deadly risks associated with the use of their products around the world. I believed that Schering had a most direct scientific and ethical responsibility to join in this research on vitamins and the prevention of cardiovascular diseases. By doing so, they could have helped millions of women taking their "Pills" - saving many from premature death from heart attacks or strokes.

But nothing could be further from the truth. After my visit at their headquarters, I never heard from them again.

This was another remarkable example of the unscrupulous conduct of the business with disease by the drug companies. Despite the "smoke screen" of running a business to improve the health of the people, the primary purpose of the drug companies is to make money from ongoing diseases. Preventing heart attacks and strokes is not in the interest of companies that sell drugs for dissolving blood clots after a heart attack has happened.

The market place for the pharmaceutical companies is the

human body and the diseases it hosts or develops. Any drugs that prevent or eradicate these diseases endanger this business; they may not be developed and become available for patients for that very reason.

During the decade-long battle towards the eradication of cardiovascular disease, I became one of the leading observers of this inscrupulous "business with diseases" by multi-billion-dollar interest groups. Among my personal experiences, the direct contact with lead researchers and executives of these companies openly ignoring their responsibility to help save lives of millions of patients was one of the most sobering and eye-opening.

I consider it my responsibility to share these experiences with you, my readers, in order to enable you to take a more objective look at the interest groups that drive the health care system. This will empower you to protect yourselves from falling victim to this "business with disease."

Despite these negative experiences with the pharmaceutical industry, all these efforts have to be regarded as another milestone in this process. Even though we did not win over one single pharmaceutical company to help disseminate this medical breakthrough, I learned two important lessons.

First, the pharmaceutical companies showed their true colors, the primary purpose for their existence is to expand their billion dollar "business with disease." The second lesson was that pharmaceutical companies will never be partners in the eradication of cardiovascular disease, one of their most lucrative sources of income. The total annual sales of cardiovascular drugs - that primarily treat the symptoms, but don't cure - has crossed the 100 billion dollar threshold.

If cardiovascular diseases were to be eradicated I needed to do it myself. With Linus's health visibly failing at age 92, it would be up to me to pick up the torch and lead this battle towards the eradication of heart disease and towards making health a human right. As difficult as it was, as high as the mountain appeared that I needed to climb, the task was clear.

MILESTONE:

Informing the Media and the Public

How vitamins became the title story

of *TIME* magazine

In April 1992, *TIME* magazine printed a cover story entitled "The Real Power of Vitamins." Suddenly, after decades of running amok against the health benefits of vitamins, this opinion shaping journal not only reported rather objectively about progress in vitamin research, but also featured it as the cover story. Of course, it was not to its disadvantage; this issue of *TIME* became the best selling issue in its history.

The event that triggered the TIME Magazine article was a conference held by the New York Academy of Sciences in February 1992 on the latest progress in vitamin research. The chances that the date of this vitamin conference was a coincidence are zero. It took place less than a year after the publication of our "Solution to the Puzzle of Cardiovascular Disease." Evidently, this recent breakthrough in the area of cardiovascular disease and vitamins triggered a frenzy of activities by distinguished scientific organizations to catch up with this development.

But it was not the scientific advances that were in the minds of the organizers or giving credit to the scientist who made these discoveries. The fact that they did not invite either Linus Pauling or me as a speaker showed that the purpose of this conference was that of a placeholder. The motto was obvious: If you can't beat them, join them; or better, try to take over the topic in order to control the public debate. The strategy was to "concede" some of the "power of vitamins" in order to prevent the public explosion of the "Eradicating Heart Disease" message. One more time, scientific organizations like the New York Academy of Sciences appeared to be part of the big "Chess Game" played by billion dollar industries. Or why was this Academy symposium the first one ever with such a heavy participation of invited media representatives? The PR effect was obviously planned.

When I accidentally found out about this conference, I decided to fly to Washington and participate not as a speaker but in the audience. The presentation on vitamins and heart disease was made by Dr. Jialal from the University of Texas. He was invited to present the antiquated theory that oxidation of cholesterol or lipoproteins would cause cardiovascular disease. It does not take a medical degree to call this bluff. Oxidation of cholesterol is - at best - a contributing factor but not the cause of cardiovascular disease. There is a simple explanation for that. If oxidation of cholesterol or other blood components were to start this disease by damaging the blood vessel wall, the deposits would develop everywhere along the cardiovascular system. Oxidized cholesterol, lipoproteins and other blood components would have contact with the wall of the arteries, capillaries and veins and would lead not only to clogging of the arteries of the heart but also of the nose, knee and even the veins. But no one has ever heard of such bizarre events as nose attacks or knee infarctions.

The scientist from Texas who gave this presentation at the New York Academy of Sciences was invited in order to put the finger in the dam of an antiquated hypothesis of cardiovascular disease. It is clear: the "oxidized-cholesterol" story keeps the cholesterol/ heart disease fallacy alive. The vitamin C/ scurvy/ heart disease connection targets the weakness of the artery wall as the primary target. This switch in therapeutic directions is not just of academic importance. In the long run it destroys a multi-billion-dollar market of cholesterol-lowering drugs.

The presentation of Dr. Jialal reminded me of someone who tried to define the medical world as being a plate at the time when its true shape had been identified as a globe. Of course, I felt challenged. My discovery had just defined the medical world as a globe and I had to fight for it!

After he had finished his presentation, I went to the floor microphone to present our new understanding about the nature of cardiovascular disease to the researchers and media representatives. In no uncertain terms, I stated in front of the research elite and the press that if he was right we would all get infarctions in the nose, ears or knees. The only rationale that could explain heart attacks as the primary cause of cardiovascular diseases was the scurvy/ heart disease connection. My contribution to this scientific debate is in the official 1992 Academy documentation of of this symposium.

After the symposium one of the participants, a scientist from Hoffman-LaRoche, approached me. "Your contribution was the only really new aspect of this whole symposium."

Apparently, the representative of *TIME* magazine who participated in this symposium felt the same. Only a few weeks later, *TIME* magazine came out in April 1992 with a title story "The Real Power Of Vitamins" and the title page prominently promised the readers to get the latest advances in vitamins and heart disease research.

But this title was misleading. Nothing inside the rather objective article on the health benefits of vitamins talked about heart disease. How could that happen? The most likely explanation was that the journalist present at the symposium of the Academy tried to report about the discovery of the scurvy-heart disease connection - after all it was news. Most likely, the "Censor-in-Chief" of *TIME* magazine pulled the plug at the last minute on this segment of the report.

What could have been the motive for such a censorship? No leading news magazine in the world is more dependent on multi-million-dollar advertising by the pharmaceuticals companies than *TIME* magazine. It was in their interest that the wildfire on the "vitamin C/ scurvy/ heart disease connection" was stopped and not further fuelled by *TIME* Magazine. But apparently, it was too late to change the cover of the magazine and remove the bold announcement on the real power of vitamins in the fight against "heart disease" from the title page. All these observations are just interesting little episodes that reveal the methods, intrigues, ruses and other maneuvers by which this battle for the eradication of heart disease is being waged.

The vitamin C/ heart disease connection had forced the largest news magazine in the world to print a cover on the objective health benefits of vitamins. Millions of vitamin consumers and thousands of health food stores could not believe the sudden shift about the health benefits of vitamins.

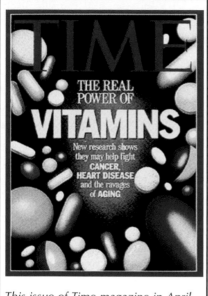

This issue of Time magazine in April 1992 became the best-selling issue in the history of the magazine.

This *TIME* article was truly a watershed event in the century. After decades of bias and boycotts against vitamins in the media, it was this *TIME* magazine article that would forever change journalism about vitamins. From then on, many epidemiological studies showing the benefits of vitamins in the prevention of heart disease and other ailments received objective reporting. Only weeks after this *TIME* article appeared, an important study by Dr. James Enstrom and his colleagues from the University of Los Angeles received national attention. This study published in *Epidemiology* showed that long-term vitamin C supplementation could reduce the rate for heart disease by half.

The available and objective media coverage about the health benefits of natural health products led to a change of public perception in favor of vitamins.

But during the first week of April 1992 another historic development took its course.

MILESTONE:

The Rath-Pauling-Manifesto

Normally, if a medical record is made, it will take years for the benefit to become available. This was not the case in the "vitamin C/ scurvy/ heart disease" connection. The key substances, vitamin C, lysine and some other essential nutrients were already available. Thus it was clear that the medical breakthrough would depend on one factor only: how fast the information about this medical advance could be disseminated to patients around the world.

After all the experiences with doctors, scientists, pharmaceutical companies and other players summarized above, I knew we needed to go directly to the people with this message. At age 92, the two-time Nobel laureate would not be around for long as a prominent supporter for this medical breakthrough. Something needed to be done quickly.

With the assistance of the Canadian *Journal of Orthomolecular Medicine,* I convinced Linus to give a keynote lecture announcing this medical breakthrough to the general public. The event was to take place in the King Edward Hotel in Toronto.

I remember sitting beside Linus Pauling in the airplane and showing him a draft of the document that would become the Rath-Pauling Manifesto. Linus was reluctant at first. I knew that he rarely chose avenues directly to the public. I reminded Linus that once before he had addressed the entire world on an issue of life and death.

In 1958, he had issued a call for a global halt to the testing of nuclear weapons in the atmosphere. Tests had led to a dramatic increase of birth defects in the United States and other countries. Within months, more than eleven thousand scientists had signed this appeal to the governments of the nuclear powers and urged them to sign a nuclear test ban treaty. Shortly thereafter, the *Partial Test Ban Treaty* was signed by the United States, the Soviet Union and other nuclear powers. In 1962, Linus Pauling received the Nobel Peace Prize for bringing about this treaty that has saved thousands of children from being born crippled.

Referring to this event four decades ago, I said "Linus, once before you called upon the entire world because so many lives were at stake. Now there is another historic situation and our responsibility is even bigger. If we don't speak out now, millions of people will suffer unnecessarily and die prematurely from heart attacks, strokes, and other preventable diseases. Later generations will ask us, what did you do when you knew it? I want to be able to say: we told the entire world!" Linus looked at me; "Let me think about it." The next morning he called me to his room in the King Edward Hotel. He had rewritten the entire "Call to Abolish Heart Disease" in his own handwriting.

The Happiest Day in the Life of a Nobel Laureate

That evening Linus gave his lecture to an audience of over 500 people, including the representative of the British Queen. The speech was well received, and the Manifesto was distributed to everyone present. After the talk, I brought Linus to his hotel room and he invited me in. Without taking off his blazer or his beret, he fell backwards onto the hotel bed and beamed. "Matthias, come here!" He took me in his arms - like a father to a son. No word was spoken - and yet everything was said in this moment. This was the day when Linus knew that his life's work would continue.

In order to improve the impact of this international call, Linus and I held a press conference in the Mark Hopkins Hotel in San Francisco on July 2, 1992. We sent press packages to all major media, TV-stations and news agencies, including copies of the publications and the manifesto. The media coverage of this historic press conference left much to be desired. The few reports in newspapers were rather biased. The journalists writing these articles clearly had not understood their responsibility for the health and lives of millions of people.

THE GOAL OF ELIMINATING

HEART DISEASE AS THE

MAJOR CAUSE OF DEATH

AND DISABILITY IS

NOW IN SIGHT!

Matthias Rath and Linus Pauling

"The elimination of heart disease is possible."
The last page of the Rath-Pauling Manifesto.

In spite of this irresponsible role of the media, the Rath-Pauling-Manifesto and this press conference became another milestone on the journey to eradicating cardiovascular disease.

Three weeks later, Linus Pauling signed a document stating that I should continue his life's work. Despite this encouraging step, I later left the Linus Pauling Institute to found my own research firm. I did this because the children of Linus Pauling - all of them at retirement age and rather skeptical about their father's interest in vitamins - made it clear that they did not wish the name of their father to be used for a campaign to eradicate heart disease.

I was unimpressed and decided to avoid a family feud. On his deathbed, he rose against his very own family and stated under oath: "There is no doubt in my mind that I thought about Dr. Rath as my successor." The Nobel laureate had acknowledged the original discoveries and transferred the ownership of the patents and other intellectual property to me in writing.

On August 19, 1994, Linus Pauling passed away. That night, shortly after 11 p.m, a journalist from the *San Francisco Chronicle* called and and asked me for a few words. I said, "Linus Pauling was a great man, and he deserves to be remembered for all the good he did for humanity."

MILESTONE

Empowering Millions of People Through Health Information

Now on my own, the first task I faced was to disseminate the information about the medical breakthrough. I decided to write a popular health book with many illustrations so the benefits of vitamins would be understandable to everyone. *Eradicating Heart Disease* and *Why Animals Don't Get Heart Attacks* were the first books at that time. Today these books are summarized in the Cellular Health Series book: *The Heart.*

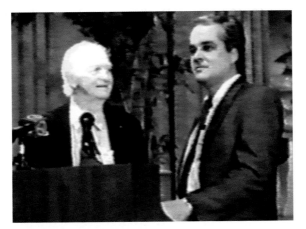

At the historic press conference on July 2, 1992, with Dr. Pauling

For people around the world these books:

- Explained for the first time in illustrated form how their cardiovascular system works.

- Revealed that cardiovascular diseases develop at the level of cells of the artery walls and the heart.

- Showed that heart attacks and strokes are not predetermined by fate but are caused by vitamin deficiencies in the cardiovascular cells.

- Empowered them to take greater responsibility for their own health with practical recommendations for natural health.

- Answered the question: "Why have I not heard about this before?" unmasking the "Business with Diseases" as the basis for the pharmaceutical industry.

Hundreds of thousands of people in Europe and elsewhere were empowered by these books to take greater responsibility for their own health. Patients took them to their doctors – many of whom were still skeptical – allowing them to win the support of their doctors for vitamin therapy and other natural health remedies.

The success of my books did not go unnoticed. During the last ten years, every major medical school, every doctors association, and even pharmaceutical companies came out with their own "self-help" health book or information brochure. The once heavily guarded fortresses of medical wisdom had been conquered. This is even more significant since this wisdom had been encoded in unintelligible languages, like Latin and Greek, in order to protect this information from becoming available to the common person.

Popular health books had been on the market before. But never before were the gatekeepers of established medicine,

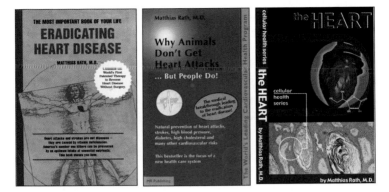

Eradicating Heart Disease
Why Animals Don't Get Heart Attacks-But People Do
Cellular Health Series: The Heart

the medical schools of Harvard, Stanford University, and the like, forced to share their information with millions of patients as they had during the last ten years. Never before did the Mayo Clinic distribute a "Health Newsletter" for the general public. Now they had to. Never before was there a course on Health and Nutrition taught at Rutgers University. Now there was. Never before did Stanford University run its own TV-Show on health issues. Now they had to - in order not to miss the train. Even the American Heart Association was forced to follow this example and published *Your Heart Manual.* But these lay books and popular brochures had one caveat: while the information about the function of the body finally had to be provided to the people, this was only a partial concession. Each chapter of these books insured that the readers were driven back into the arms of the ravenous "Business with Diseases."

My books were fundamentally different. They empowered their readers to abandon the shackles of dependencies of the "Business with Diseases" and liberate themselves by understanding the principles of cellular health.

In the fifth century B.C., Hipppocrates, the father of all doctors, made his students swear to keep the secrets of medicine from their patients. This oath is still taken at many medical schools around the world!

My books helped patients and people around the world articulate the urge for more health information. They are no longer willing to remain uninformed about their own health and be led like sheep from one disease to the next.

This "liberation of health" was another important milestone to eradicating heart disease as well as other common health problems.

MILESTONE

Cellular Health and Cellular Medicine - Foundations of a New Health Care

One of the most important milestones was the development of Cellular Health and Cellular Medicine. After the discovery that atheroclerosis, heart attacks and strokes are primarily caused by vitamin deficiency the question was: What about the other common health problems associated with cardiovascular diseases, such as high blood pressure, heart failure, etc.?

There were studies about certain essential nutrients reporting about health benefits. Dr. Folkers showed the benefits of Coenzyme Q-10 in heart failure patients; Drs. England and Turlapaty studied magnesium in patients with irregular heartbeat, and so on, but these were isolated observations. The following lack of understanding prevented earlier completion of the entire picture of Celllar Medicine:

- The fact that diseases develop at the level of cells was ignored, and it was not understood that the primary cause of cellular malfunction is a deficiency of vitamins and other essential nutrients required for cell fuel.

- The fact that the heart is the motor of the body and that for proper function it requires regular refilling of biological fuel just like your car needs gasoline. Since this basic problem had never been properly identified by conventional medicine, the cells of the heart and the artery walls of millions of people literally ran dry of cell fuel.

- As the direct result of this, lack of information and knowledge, heart attacks, strokes, high blood pressure, heart failure and other forms of cardiovascular disease that develop as a result of cellular energy deficiency continue to spread like epidemics.

· Moreover, it had not been understood that the pumping heart muscles do not just use *one* individual vitamin as fuel. They need regular replenishing of *many* vitamins, minerals, trace elements and amino acids. This lack of understanding also explains why clinical studies were done usually involving one nutrient rather than the whole range of vitamins and other biochemical cofactors for cellular energy production.

· Finally, it had not been understood by conventional medicine that the treatment of isolated symptoms of CVD such as high blood pressure, heart failure or angina pectoris would be insufficient as long as the lack of vitamins and other bioenergy molecules is not replenished.

I still remember the day when the thought of Cellular Medicine struck me. For some time, my brain had been constantly working on the discoveries, sorting new thoughts and assembling them in an orderly fashion. The vitamin programs I had developed resulted in many letters from patients reporting health improvements, from lowered blood pressure to the disappearance of angina pectoris and edema.

Then it suddenly struck me. I realized that today's most common diseases related to the cardiovascular system must have the same cause: deficiency of cellular bioenergy. Heart failure was not the result of a lack of Coenzym Q -10 alone but of a range of cellular energy cofactors.

I immediately realized the general nature and the significance of this discovery for human health. Back in the office of our research firm, I called my colleagues and we had a little toast on this discovery.

Never before had anyone proposed such far-reaching conclusions and defined the deficiency of essential nutrients as the *primary* cause of today's most common diseases. The new understanding of Cellular Health would help millions of patients and eventually reduce these diseases to a fraction of today's numbers.

Later it also became clear to me that it was no coincidence that the most wide-spread diseases of our time had such a simple explanation as vitamin deficiency. In the interest of the multi-billion dollar pharmaceutical drug market, these common health problems were deliberately mystified. Diagnostic code names were used to mask vitamin deficiency as the true nature of these diseases.

The majority of patients with high blood pressure were diagnosed with the cover term "essential hypertension." Most patients with heart failure had "idiopathic" cardiomyopathy, and most patients with irregular heartbeat went under the diagnosis "paroxysmal" arrhythmia. The terms "essential", "idiopathic" and "paroxysmal" are Greek and Latin terms for the same message: "cause unknown."

While millions of patients are led to believe that they have been precisely diagnosed, they received the encoded stamp: "We don't know the cause of your disease." Conventional medicine ignores this mass deception because it is built on treating *symptoms*, e.g. lowering high blood pressure - not curing it. For treating the symptoms with a pharmaceutical drug, e.g. a blood pressure lowering drug, the doctors do not need to know the cause of the disease. To keep the drug companies happy, they need only to fill out prescription forms for the symptom drugs.

We must realize that this deception towards millions of patients is a precondition of the multi-billion dollar pharmaceutical "business with disease." Preventing, curing and eradicating diseases are all damaging to the "business with diseases." Despite the PR efforts that portray the drug companies as benefactors to mankind, they seek - like any other business - to expand their markets. And their market places are human bodies

Now we understand why today's pharmaceutically oriented medicine uses code names for the most common diseases: No one needs to know; no one should ask uncomfortable questions; and the billion dollar "business with disease" can go on.

However, only patients and people "who don't know" will tolerate this deception and pay up to one third of their income for a medicine that merely treats symptoms.

This deplorable situation further underlines the importance of of Cellular Medicine as the foundation of a new health care system in the United States and elsewhere.

FURTHER MILESTONES

- IN THE USA -

- The next milestone in the U.S. was the development of a basic Cellular Health Program that would allow people to benefit immediately from this medical breakthrough. Towards that end I developed a basic Cellular Health Program, including the natural ingredients that had been patented for the natural prevention of cardiovascular disease.

- Subsequently we conducted a clinical study with coronary heart disease patients with this Cellular Health program. Using the latest diagnostic technology, Ultrafast Computed Tomography, the so-called "Mammogram of the Heart" we could show that without vitamin supplementation, the deposits in the coronary arteries normally grow by 44% each year. With a defined vitamin program, the further growth of these deposits could be stopped in its early stages. In some cases, reversal and complete disappearance of existing deposits was documented.

- From 1994 to 1996, I gave lectures, radio and TV interviews throughout the United States, promoting this medical breakthrough and my books. Tens of thousands were reached by the lectures, millions by the radio and TV shows. The discovery of the scurvy/heart disease connection and the news that heart disease can eventually be eradicated reached doctor's offices across America.

- Following this information and education campaign, the floodgates of established medicine were opening. Vitamins and essential nutrients entered conventional medicine.

- The *Journal of the American Medical Association* (JAMA), published an article on the use of antioxidant vitamins as a basic treatment for coronary heart disease.

- In October, 1995, the leading medical schools in America established departments of nutritional medicine to pro-

Breathtaking Perspective of Cellular Medicine

- Reveals to millions of patients the true nature of today's most common diseases - vitamin deficiency;

- Empowers millions of people to take responsibility for their own health and help prevent these health problems in an effective, safe and affordable way;

- Delivers the scientific grounds for terminating the "business with disease" and for making health a human right, available to everyone - just like education.

Cause of disease unknown

	Before Cellular Medicine	With Cellular Medicine
Heart Attacks	80%	→ 5%
Strokes	80%	→ 5%
High Blood Pressure	90%	→ 5%
Heart Failure	90%	→ 1%
Irregular Heart Beat	70%	→ 5%
Adult Diabetes	95%	→ 1%

Each of these reductions accounts for millions of lives saved.

vide to future generations of doctors with a basic understanding about the health benefits of vitamins and other essential nutrients.

- The National Institutes of Health (NIH) gave multi-million dollar research grants to ten leading research institutions in America, among them Stanford University, to study alternative treatments, including vitamin therapy.

- In patient brochures, self-help books, and community newsletters, the leading medical schools, including Harvard University, started to recommend vitamins as basic health measures.

FURTHER MILESTONES

- IN EUROPE -

- Following the initial information campaign in the U.S., I decided to bring this important health message to Europe. This was even more significant, since the people in Europe lived in Medieval Times with respect to vitamins and nutritional supplements. While in the U.S., every second person was supplementing their diet, these numbers in Europe were below five percent, in some countries below one percent. The primary responsibility for this disastrous state of affairs was the European pharmaceutical companies who had demonized vitamins or simply outlawed them as "drugs." With medicine heavily lobbied by the pharmaceutical drug manufacturers, German law defined a pill containing 500 milligrams of vitamin C as a prescription drug! Selling these vitamin C "drugs" was considered a criminal offense.

Luckily, the dogs, lambs, goats and sheep of Germany all

smiled at the myopia of the German government: these animals produced 30 times that amount of vitamin C every day in their bodies - without waiting for any prescription or standing in line at the pharmacy and without asking the German government for legislative permission.

- One of the next milestones in Europe was the development of a comprehensive Cellular Health program. It met the additional nutritional needs of people with certain health conditions, including high blood pressure, heart failure, diabetes, high cholesterol levels, circulatory problems, increased susceptibility to infections, and others. The immediate success of these programs confirmed the importance of Cellular Medicine as the basis for approaching a multitude of health problems at their roots. Today our Cellular Health programs are the leading nutritional health programs across Europe.

- The next milestone was the clinical testing of these programs in pilot studies. The results of these pilot studies with our Cellular Health programs can be obtained from our Website at www.dr-rath-research.org.

- The next milestone was the decision by one of the leading health insurance companies in Germany to reimburse the costs for the Cellular Health programs. This decision did not come easily. The health benefits had to be documented by an attending doctor, but it was a wise decision. Economically the health insurance companies and HMO's gain by supporting this medical breakthrough. With the help of Cellular Health programs, effective health care can now be provided at a fraction of previous costs.

Of course, these milestones are but a few of the events that took place while disseminating the "eradicating heart disease" message on a global level. A more comprehensive report is in preparation, and I am confident that scientific historians will join in to elucidate this historic mission for a broad audience.

The milestones and accomplishments summarized in this chapter did not come easily. At every step I met boycotts, intimidations, legal and regulatory threats, personal attacks and just about every offense one can imagine from an industry that is fighting to artificially stabilize a multi-billion market of cardiovascular drugs.

In the following chapter, I will document the most important of these obstacles to be surmounted to bring this process forward to this day.

Roadblocks

of the Medical Breakthrough

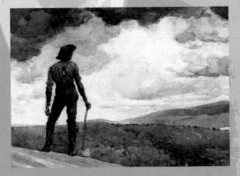

"There is no more delicate matter to take in hand, nor more dangerous to conduct, than to stand up as a leader in the introduction of change.

For he who innovates will have as enemies all those who are well off under the existing order of things and only luke warm supporters in those who might be better of under the new system."

Niccolo Machiavelli,
Advisor to the Medici Court A.D. 1513

The medical breakthrough of the scurvy/heart disease connection and the foundation of Cellular Medicine was such a threat to the interests of the drug companies that they reacted immediately.

One faction embarked on an effort to ban by law the dissemination of this medical breakthrough and by making vitamins prescription drugs.

The other group of companies embarked on taking economic advantage of this breakthrough by conspiring in criminal price fixing practices.

The following pages summarize these historic events.

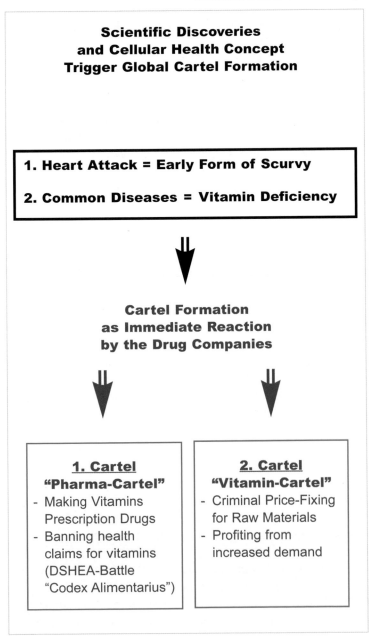

**Scientific Discoveries
and Cellular Health Concept
Trigger Global Cartel Formation**

1. Heart Attack = Early Form of Scurvy

2. Common Diseases = Vitamin Deficiency

**Cartel Formation
as Immediate Reaction
by the Drug Companies**

**1. Cartel
"Pharma-Cartel"**
- Making Vitamins
  Prescription Drugs
- Banning health
  claims for vitamins
  (DSHEA-Battle
  "Codex Alimentarius")

**2. Cartel
"Vitamin-Cartel"**
- Criminal Price-Fixing
  for Raw Materials
- Profiting from
  increased demand

Triggering the Vitamin Freedom Act (DSHEA) of 1994

Immediately following publication of the scurvy/heart disease connection in 1992, the U.S. Food and Drug Administration (FDA) started a public campaign with the goal of making vitamins prescription drugs. While every vitamin consumer and every health food store in America was outraged about those efforts, no one asked the decisive question: What triggered this shameless attack on the freedom of the American people and on their right to choose their own health care? Why was it the fiercest FDA attack on nutritional supplements thus far?

The answer is provided in this book. The outrageous action by the FDA was neither a coincidence nor a long-term plan. It was a direct and deliberate reaction of the pharmaceutical industry to the discovery of the scurvy/heart disease connection. The drug manufacturer executives knew that if vitamins are the solution to the cardiovascular epidemic, a prescription drug market of over 100 billion dollars annually would collapse.

But why did the FDA lead the attack? Thomas Moore revealed in his book *Deadly Medicine* that most of the FDA experts were also on the payroll of pharmaceutical companies. This explained why this federal agency did not act on behalf of the interests of millions of Americans but on behalf of those special interests representing the "business with disease."

But millions of Americans said no to these unethical and transparent plans of the Pharmaceutical Cartel. In August 1994, the U.S. Congress unanimously passed legislation preserving free access to vitamins and other essential nutri-

The Worst Defeat of the Pharmaceutical Industry

To protect their markets of pharamceutical drugs, the drug manufacturers wanted to ban all health information in relation to vitamins and make them prescription drugs. It was clear to the drug companies that hundreds of millions of Americans who had been enjoying free access to vitamins over decades would not understand why vitamins should suddenly become pre-scription drugs. Thus, the pharmceutical companies abused the FDA to present a Public Relation camouflage to the American people and make their unethical plans palatable and acceptable:

- **"Consumer Protection"** In a large-scale public relations campaign, the FDA, on behalf of the Pharma-Cartel, tried to make millions of Americans believe that vitamins and other natural therapies had to become prescription items in order to protect them from "overdosing." That house of cards collapsed when the following U.S. statistics became public: From 1983 to 1990, not a single death resulted from intake of vitamins, amino acids, or other natural products. In contrast, during the same period, almost one million Americans died as a consequence of taking prescription drugs that had been approved by the FDA!

- **"Internationalization"** The second cover-name under which the FDA and the Cartel tried to limit free access to vitamins was the alleged necessity for internationally unified guidelines for vitamins. Perhaps with their eyes on Germany and other European countries, where one-gram vitamin C is defined as a prescription drug and where amino acids are on the "black list," these special interest groups tried to turn nutritional medicine back to medieval times.

But the American people were neither interested in "consumer protection" from vitamins nor in "internationalization." In the "largest movement since the Vietnam War" (Newsweek) the American people, through their political representatives, secured Vitamin Freedom and defeated the FDA and the Pharma-Cartel.

ents. The Dietary Supplement Health and Education Act (DSHEA) was one of the historic victories of the American people.

How could this attack by the drug companies and the FDA on vitamins be turned into a victory for vitamin freedom? Many contributed to this historic success, but most important were those millions of Americans who made it unmistakably clear to their political representatives that they will have free access to their vitamins today – and in the future!

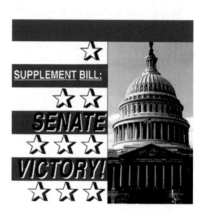

My first book *Eradicating Heart Disease* contained an Open Letter to the President. As an Open Letter, the primary addressees were the American people, to empower them to take a stand on this important issue. Health food store owners informed me that copies of this "Open Letter to the President" were picked up in their stores "like hot cakes," together with petitions to political representatives to halt the plans of the FDA. Thus, the medical breakthrough in vitamin and heart disease research that triggered this battle also became a contributing factor to winning it.

Codex Alimentarius -
Effort to Ban Natural Health Information World Wide

Following the loss of the battle to make vitamins prescription items in the U.S., the pharmaceutical industry regrouped and formed a cartel at the international level. They started a worldwide campaign to outlaw all preventive and therapeutic health information about vitamins and other natural therapies. Abusing the United Nation's *Codex Alimentarius* (food standards) Commission they are trying to ban any natural health claims in all UN member countries; that is, worldwide. The decisive Committee on nutritional supplements is headed by the German government. No wonder Germany exports more pharmaceutical products than any other nation.

To make sure these controversial plans would pass in countries where resistance would be strong, such as the U.S., the Cartel threatened international trade sanctions in case of non-compliance. If the people and the governments of the United Kingdom, the United States, Canada, Australia or any other country refused to accept vitamins as prescription drugs, they would be faced with UN trade sanctions. With this strategy, the Pharma-Cartel tried to twist the arms of the entire corporate world, and at the same time, declared war on the health interests of millions of people.

The cartel moved fast. By the end of 1996, the Pharma-Cartel's *Codex* plans had already reached Stage Five of an eight-stage process within the United Nations. Disguised as "consumer protection" these unconscionable plans were about to be recommended to the UN General Assembly for adoption. This was the situation until June 21, 1997.

On that day, I decided to confront these interest groups on their home turf. I knew that I would be representing the health interests of millions of people. I gave a speech to 3,400 people in the city hall of Chemnitz, Germany. I revealed the connection between the *Codex* Cartel, the German Government and its roots in the history of those German chemical and pharmaceutical companies who were the profiteers of World War II and the Holocaust. With a view on the devastating consequences of the *Codex* plans for global human health, I stated:

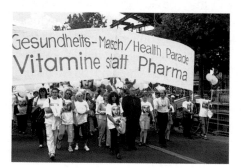

More than 3,000 people demonstrated in Berlin against Codex Alimentarius. More than 500,000 protest letters reached the Codex Commission members. The unethical plans could not go through.

"Twice in this century, indescribable worldwide suffering and death originated from Germany. This must not happen a third time."

This speech was immediately distributed via the Internet. Thousands of audio and videotapes followed.

But the cartel did not give up. The most recent meeting of the Codex Alimentarius Commission took place in June 2000 in Berlin. The aim of the meeting was again a worldwide ban on health information concerning natural therapies. To camouflage its activities, the pharmaceutical cartel and its political accomplices hid in the "Federal Office for Consumer Health Protection" (BgVV), hermetically sealed behind barbed wire.

On the eve of this conference, we held a health conference with 2000 participants and a rally through the city of Berlin and at the site of the meeting.

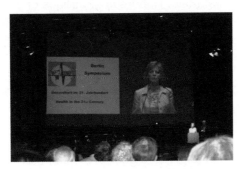

Codex Alimentarius is a reaction of the pharmaceutical industry to the break-throughs in natural health. At our confer-ence "Health in the 21st Century", patients, doctors and scientists summa-rized this breakthrough.
Above Dr. Aleksandra Niedzwiecki, U.S.A.

Most important, more than half a million protest letters were sent from our website to the *Codex* Delegates alerting them not to follow the German delegation.

As a result of this international protest, the debate in the *Codex* Commission was so controversial that the plans of the pharmaceutical cartel - once again - did not pass.

We had accomplished a victory in the name of the people of the world and for the benefit of their health.

Busting the Vitamin Cartel

On May 20, 1999, the media bomb detonated. The multinational corporations Hoffmann-LaRoche, BASF, Rhône-Poulenc, among other multinational pharmaceutical companies, admitted to forming a "Vitamin-Cartel" to fix the price of vitamin raw materials. Hundreds of millions of people worldwide were defrauded for almost a decade and had to pay higher vitamin prices because of these criminal activities. The U.S. Justice Department declared that this Vitamin Cartel was the largest cartel ever discovered and named it an economic "conspiracy." Roche, BASF and the other cartel members agreed to pay almost a billion dollars in fines.

While the magnitude of these fines made headlines around the world, the events that triggered the formation of this criminal cartel remained obscure. Until now. The background of this illegal Vitamin Cartel is the scientific breakthrough documented in this book in relation to vitamins and prevention of cardiovascular disease. In 1990, I informed the Swiss multinational pharmaceutical company Hoffmann-La Roche about these discoveries. On June 2, 1990, I sent the summary of the discovery that heart attacks and strokes are – similar to scurvy – the result of vitamin C deficiency to Prof. Jürgen Drews, head of Roche research worldwide and member of its executive board.

Roche is the world's leading manufacturer of vitamin C raw material. The Roche executives realized immediately that my discovery would boost their international demand for vitamin C and create a multi-billion dollar market for vitamin C and other vitamins. In order to extract further information from me, the executives of Hoffmann-La Roche signed a confidentiality agreement and invited me to present the new understanding of heart disease at their global headquarter in

June 4, 1990

CONFIDENTIAL

Professor Jürgen Drews
Hoffmann-La Roche & Co. AG
Grenzacherstrasse 122
Basel
CH-4058 Baselstadt
Switzerland

Dear Professor Drews:

Following our conversation on the vitamin C-related atherosclerosis research we send you today the concept of this work. ... ... The implications of this concept for human health are obvious. Our research promises to provide important missing links on the cellular and molecular level to prove the role of vitamin C on prevention and therapy for cardiovascular disease and other diseases. Beside animal studies conducted, we have obtained preliminary data from patients in support of this concept. If further evidence can be provided, we foresee a several-fold increase in the preventive and therapeutic use of vitamin C.

As a next step we suggest that further evidence should be provided on various research levels. We could offer links to other research labs and clinical centers interested in this field.

We are convinced of the mutual benefit of our discovery and its scientific and commercial impacts. We are looking forward to your reply.

Sincerely,

Dr. Matthias Rath

MR:mb

⟨Roche⟩

F. HOFFMANN-LA ROCHE AG

Law Department

Your Ref.: MR:
Our Ref.: StA/Co-mb
Direct Dialling: 061 688 58 66   Basel, June 18, 1990

Agreement of Confidentiality

Dear Dr. Rath,

We are refering to the draft Agreement of Confidentiality of May 25, 1990, already signed by you.

May we kindly ask you to send us a second original of the Agreement of Confidentialty already duly signed by you. After full execution of both originals, we shall return to you one original and keep the other one for our files.

Yours sincerely,

F.HOFFMANN-LA ROCHE Ltd

Prof. J. Drews   Dr. C. Conti

CH-4002 Basel, Schweiz
Telephon 061-6881111
Telex 962292/965542 hir ch
Telefax 061-6919391/6919600

F.HOFFMANN-LA ROCHE LTD
CH-4002 Basel, Switzerland
Telephone 061-6881111
Telex 962292/965542 hir ch
Telefax 061-6919391/6919600

F.HOFFMANN-LA ROCHE SA
CH-4002 Bâle, Suisse
Téléphone 061-6881111
Télex 962292/965542 hir ch
Téléfax 061-6919391/6919600

Basel, Switzerland. However, Roche decided not to promote this medical breakthrough, despite the fact that they acknowledged it as a breakthrough. The reasons came in writing: Roche did not want to finance the dissemination of this understanding of heart disease for all their competitors and they did not want to compete with other in-house pharmaceutical drug developments, such as cholesterol-lowering drugs.

Thus, while they refused to promote this medical break-through that could have saved millions of lives, these phar-maceutical companies turned around and decided to conspire in the form of a vitamin cartel in order to take the advantage of this medical breakthrough anyway. Roche conspired with BASF, Rhone-Poulenc, Takeda and other manufacturers of vitamin raw materials in criminal price fixing. The profits these companies made from their criminal practices are estimated to be over 100 billion dollars over the past ten years. Compared to that, the fines these companies had to pay are inconsequential.

Not only should the U.S. government receive compensation for the damage these companies have done, vitamin companies, and above all, consumers worldwide, should sue these companies in class action lawsuits. This is even more urgent, since these companies have twice harmed millions of people. First, they refused to promote and disseminate the live-saving information on the use of vitamins in order to prevent heart disease. Second, they caused financial dam-age to literally every vitamin consumer on earth.

My correspondence with the Roche executives also proves the statements by Hoffmann-La Roche as a lie that the lead-ership of Roche did not know about these criminal activities.

The opposite is now clear: The executives of Roche, BASF, Rhône-Poulenc and others not only knew about these crimes, they were the organizers. The responsible managers should be hold accountable for their actions.

Today everyone can call those companies and their leaders criminals who distinguish themselves from a street robber only by the magnitude of their crimes. The criminal activities of this vitamin cartel have opened the eyes of millions of people further to the "business with disease" maintained by major drug companies.

A Breathtaking Perspective

There is no doubt: The turn from the second into the third millennium coincides with a change in health care worldwide. Millions of people are waking up and realizing that they have become dependent on a false health care system that was little more than an illusion.

In ever increasing numbers, patients and health professionals alike are taking advantage of the fact that the most common diseases of our time can be effectively prevented and treated by vitamins and other essential nutrients.

With the help of vitamin research and Cellular Medicine, these patients have regained a life that is worth living. Many thousands of these patients in Europe, America, and all other continents are living proof that a new health care system has already become reality.